GLOSSARY FOR RADIOLOGIC TECHNOLOGISTS

GLOSSARY FOR RADIOLOGIC TECHNOLOGISTS

Patricia A. Myers, R.T.(R), FASRT
*Director of Education
Montefiore Hospital
School of Radiography
Pittsburgh, Pennsylvania*

Therese A. Martin, R.T.(R)
*Chief Radiologic Technologist
Presbyterian-University Hospital
Department of Radiology
Pittsburgh, Pennsylvania*

PRAEGER

PRAEGER SPECIAL STUDIES • PRAEGER SCIENTIFIC

Library of Congress Cataloging in Publication Data

Myers, Patricia A
   Glossary for radiologic technologists.

   1. Radiography, Medical--Dictionaries.
2. Radiology, Medical--Dictionaries. 3. Medical
technology--Dictionaries. I. Martin, Therese A.,
joint author. II. Title. [DNLM: 1. Technology,
Radiologic--Dictionaries. WN13 M996g]
RC78.M92   616.07'572'03   80-20917
ISBN 0-03-057584-2

Published in 1981 by Praeger Publishers
CBS Educational and Professional Publishing
A Division of CBS, Inc.
521 Fifth Avenue, New York, New York 10175 U.S.A.

© 1981 by Praeger Publishers

All rights reserved

123456789 145 987654321

Printed in the United States of America

dedicated to
OUR PARENTS

PREFACE

It is obvious to anyone who has ever experienced a loss of memory of a term or phrase that a text such as this might have been useful. Many new words defined here will prove of value to radiographers in management, education, and staff, as well as to student trainees, radiologists, and those working in the radiographic field.

The preparation of the text has been aided significantly by the contributions of many individuals. We would especially like to thank John McChesney of the Picker Corporation, Sandra Yurko and Michael Murphy of Montefiore Hospital, and to express our sincere appreciation to Joanne Siksa of Presbyterian-University Hospital for typing the technical material. We would also like to thank Robert Roche, Siemens Corporation; David Veltz, Eastman Kodak Company; George Kalinyak, Xonics Medical Systems; Russ Hannan, EMI Medical Inc.; Robert Hartman, E.I. duPont de Nemours; Harold Barras, The Evans Sherratt Company; Denise Basara, Catherine Carrell, and Lisa Leonard, Presbyterian-University Hospital; Margaret Eddy, Marjorie Hunt, and Cathy Hilty, Montefiore Hospital; John Garber, General Electric Corporation; Dick Inglese, Mallinkrodt; Roy Getz, Winthrop; Joycelyn Champagne, Westmoreland Hospital; Valeria Garbinski Spero and Bernice L. Szepucha.

For their kind tolerance, we are grateful to the staff of the Radiology Department at Presbyterian-University Hospital, especially Francine M. Gardner, Evonne A. Scheller, Janet Hosper, and Loretta Hanwell; and to the students and staff of the Radiology Department at Montefiore Hospital, as well.

Last, but by no means least, we thank Bette Midler for her musical inspiration and the realization that "you got to have friends!"

CONTENTS

	Page
Preface	vii
Glossary	1
Abbreviations	165
Terminology of Radiographic Examinations (procedures)	171
Electrical Symbols	181
X-ray Circuit	187
Weights and Measures	189
References	193

GLOSSARY FOR RADIOLOGIC TECHNOLOGISTS

GLOSSARY

abberation
An undesirable characteristic of a lens or optical system. It prevents the lens from providing an exact reproduction of the original subject by degrading or distorting the image.

abrasion marks
Marks produced in the emulsion of an x-ray film by rubbing.

absorb
To take into the skin or body tissue.

absorbed dose
The quantity of absorbed radiation energy that is measured in rad; it is that energy that is taken out of the x-ray beam by an absorbing material.

absorbed dose rate
The dose per unit of time; measured in rads per unit time.

absorption
The process by which radiation imparts some or all of its energy to another material through which it may pass.

absorption coefficient
A small decrease in the intensity of the x-ray beam per unit thickness, per unit mass, or per atom absorber.

absorption unsharpness
This is caused by the absorption of the x-rays by the object being radiographed. The resulting interstructural geometric image is unsharp. Sometimes referred to as *subject unsharpness*.

absorption x-ray spectrum
That part of an x-ray beam which is not absorbed on passage through an absorber. Also referred to as remnant radiation.

acceleration
The rate at which the velocity of a body changes.

accelerator (particle)
A device that accelerates charged subatomic particles to very great energies. These particles may be used for direct medical irradiation, producing x-rays and neutrons, and for basic physical research. Medical units include linear accelerators, Van de Graff units, betatrons, and cyclotrons. Also called *particle accelerator* and *atom smasher*.

accessory
The additional part or assembly that contributes to the effectiveness of a piece of equipment without changing its basic function.

acetic acid
Found in the fixer; its purposes are to neutralize the alkali still remaining on the film and provide optimum medium for fixer and hardener.

a.c. generator
A device that changes mechanical energy to electrical energy.

acoustic impedance, ultrasound
Ratio of pressure to particle velocity.

a.c. power supply
A power supply that provides one or more a.c. output voltages, such as an a.c. generator or transformer. This type of power supplies the energy for the main switch of the x-ray circuit.

actinic radiation
That part of the electromagnetic radiation that can affect photographic film emulsion; far beyond the wavelength range of ultraviolet and visible light.

activated water
Water that has absorbed ionizing radiation.

activation
The process of inducing radioactivity by bombardment with neutrons or other types of radiation; and the process of adding liquid to a manufactured cell or battery to make it operative.

active layer, intensifying screen
The thin, smooth, abrasion-resistant coating of intensifying screens. It seals the screen against moisture, preventing warping.

active trace
That part of the television scanning system actually utilized to reproduce the subject.

activity
An expression or term for *radioactivity*.

actual focal spot
That area of the target that is always larger than the effective focal size. It is the area of the anode upon which the electrons strike. See illustration.

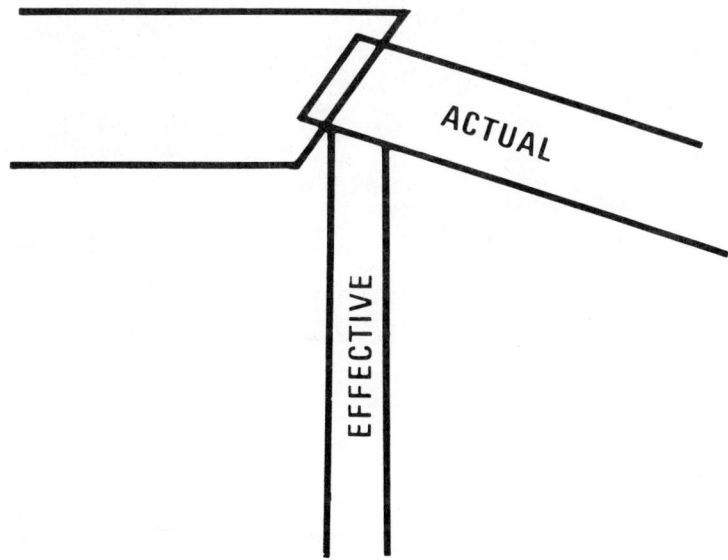

Actual Focal Spot   The actual area of the target in which the electrons strike. The effective area of the target from which primary radiation stems.

acute exposure
An intense, short exposure to ionizing radiation.

a.c. voltage
Alternating voltage.

adaptation (dark adaptation)
The adaptation of the eye to vision in the dark. Adaptation is not to be confused with accommodation, which refers to the adjustment of the eye for various distances.

added filter (filtration)
Usually referring to 2mm aluminum added to the inherent filter of a diagnostic beam for the primary purpose of filtering out soft rays having none of the penetrating characteristics. See illustration.

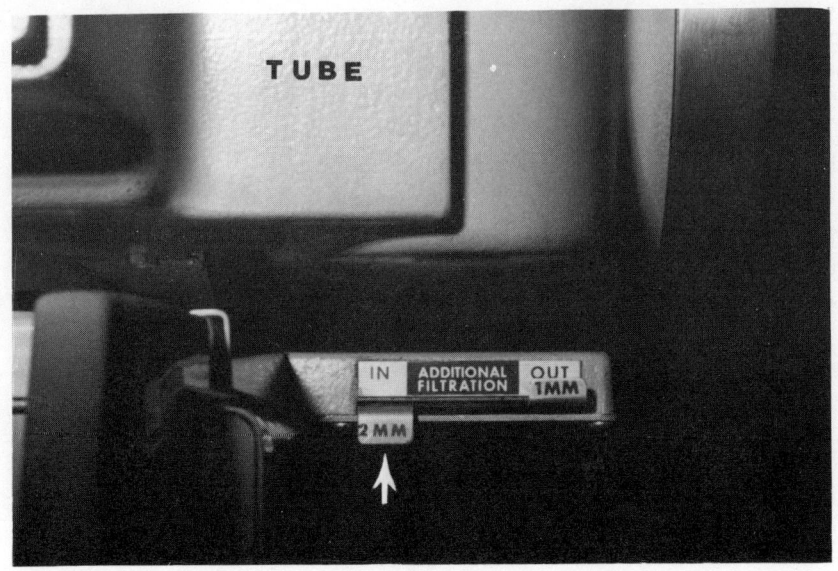

Added Filter (Filtration)

adjustable resistor
See *choke coil* and/or *rheostat*.

adjustable transformer
See *autotransformer*.

Adrian-Crooks type cassette
The cassette contains a copper step wedge, an intensifying screen, and a light absorber. The copper step wedge yields a given penetration value; the intensifying screen is not covered by the step wedge and the light from this area passes through the light absorber before reaching the film and reducing an exposure. The penetration through the light absorber remains constant and does not change with Kv.P. This area of the film is a reference density that corresponds to a known penetration value. The components of the cassette measure x-ray penetration for the purpose of determining Kv.P.

afterglow
See *phosphorescence*.

age fog
Mottled or uniform fogging due to outdated film or films stored under conditions of too high temperature and excessive humidity.

air core transformer
The simplest type of transformer consisting of two highly insulated coils of wire parallel to each other. See illustration.

Air Core Transformer

air dose
The x-ray dose in roentgens at a point in free air, including only the radiation of the primary beam and that scattered from surrounding air, measured by Victoreen R-meter. See illustration.

air gap technique
A radiographic technique used to filter out secondary and scatter radiation by placing the patient approximately six inches back from the x-ray film during the exposure. The six-inch distance from the patient to the film will act as a filter. See illustration.

air-wall ionization chamber
Used for x-ray and gamma radiation, an "air equivalent" chamber in which the materials of the wall and of the electrodes are of a substance essentially equivalent to that in a free air ionization chamber.

algorithm, CT
The specific mathematical formulas used to define the relationship between raw scanner data and processed (final) data.

alkaline
Relating to alkali, opposite reaction of acid. pH above 7, which is neutral. See *pH*.

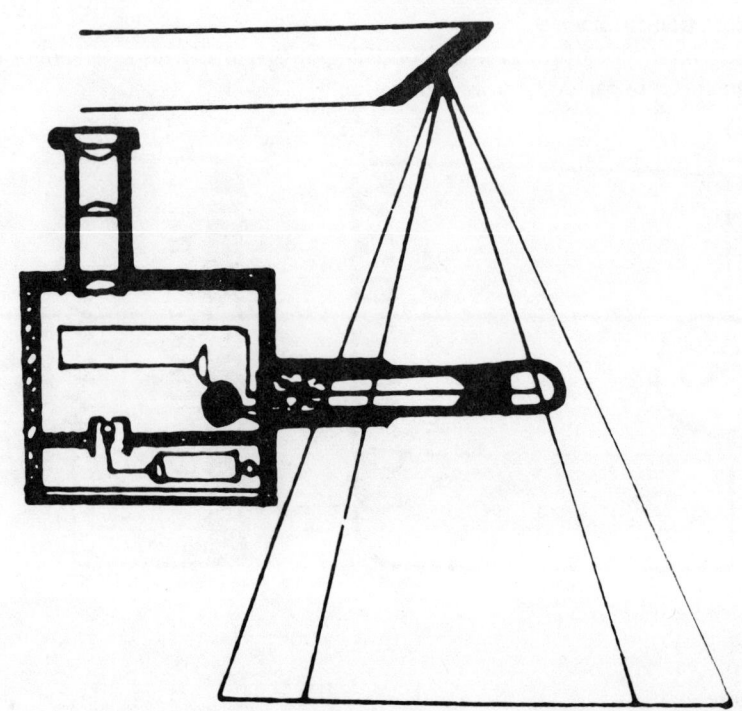

Air Dose Victoreen R-meter measuring air dose

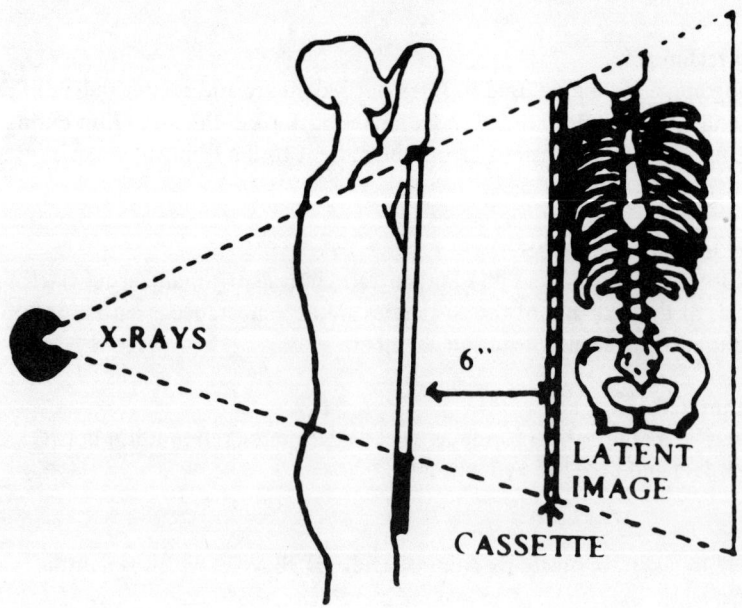

Air Gap Technique

alloy
A metal composed of two or more metals.

alnico
An alloy consisting chiefly of aluminum, nickel, and cobalt, having high retentivity. Used to make permanent magnets, as required for strong magnetic fields.

alpha
The ratio of radioactive capture to fission cross section for a fissionable element.

alpha decay
The radioactive transformation that occurs when an alpha particle is emitted by a nuclide. The decay product is a new nuclide having a mass number of four units smaller and an atomic number of two units smaller than the original nuclide.

alpha particle
The positively charged nucleus of a helium atom having two protons and two neutrons. It is emitted spontaneously from radioactive substances in their change from one element into another.

alpha radiation
Rays merging from radioactive atoms of fast moving particles. A synonym for *alpha particles*.

alternating current (a.c.)
The flow of electrons first, in one direction (1/120 sec.) and second, in the opposite direction (1/120 sec.). Each 1/120 second is referred to as an *impulse*, *pulse*, or *alternation*.

alternating voltage
Voltages that are continually varying in value and reversing their direction at regular intervals. Also called *a-c voltage*.

alternation
One-half cycle of alternating current; one alternation lasts 1/120 second. Also called an *impulse* or *pulsation*.

alternator
A machine that generates an alternating voltage when its armature or field is rotated by a motor, an engine, or other means.

aluminum
Symbol *Al*. A lightweight nonmagnetic material having the atomic number of 13. Widely used for radiographic filters, penetrometers, and electronic equipment. See *added filter*.

aluminum equivalent
The thickness of aluminum affording the same attenuation, under specified condition, as the material in question.

aluminum filter
See *added filter*.

aluminum wedge
See *penetrometer*.

alum "Tans" (chrome or potassium)
"Tans" or hardens the gelatin in the film emulsion. Protects the emulsion from scratches and is found in fixer.

ambient
The natural or inherent environment in which some event or activity is to take place.

ambient temperature
The temperature of the air surrounding the heated parts of an electric circuit.

ammeter
An instrument or meter which is placed in the series of an electrical circuit to measure amperage.

ammonium thiosulfate (fix)
Liquid fixer that clears the film by dissolving unexposed, undeveloped silver bromides.

A mode (amplitude modulation)
A method of acoustic echo display in which time is represented along the horizontal axis and echo amplitude (strength) is displayed along the vertical axis.

amperage
See *ampere*.

ampere
A unit of electrical current. The practical unit of electric current. A voltage of one volt will send a current of one ampere through a resistance of one ohm.

amphoteric material
The capability of reacting chemically either as an acid or as a base under the condition of a different pH factor. Gelatin of film emulsion is an amphoteric material.

amplification
As related to radiation detection instruments, the process (gas, electronics, or both) by which ionization effects are magnified to a degree suitable for their measurement.

amplifier
Brightness of a fluoroscopic image. See *image intensifier*.

amplitude
The distance the x-ray tube travels during the exposure of tomography radiography or any body section x-ray equipment. The longer the tube travels, the thinner the cut. See *fulcrum*.

amplitude, electrical
The range from crest to valley over which the sine wave varies.

analog, CT
The representation of numerical quantities by physical variables such as translation, rotation, voltage, and resistance. In *CT* technology, the detector's electrical analog output is the variable that retains a proportional relationship with the x-ray beam strength.

analyzer
A testing instrument used to measure voltages and currents for electronic equipment.

anechoic
The property of being echo free. A clear cyst is anechoic.

angstrom (Å)
A unit of wavelength of x-ray and other radiation. One angstrom is 10^{-8} centimeter. The electromagnetic spectrum units are measured in angstroms. Diagnostic radiation useful range is from .1Å to .5Å but all x-rays occur in a wide range from .04Å to 1000Å.

angulation of anode
Standard diagnostic tube angle 10° to 17° vertical. See illustration. Therapy tube 45°. See illustration.

anion
A negative ion that goes to the positive pole or anode in an electrochemical solution (battery).

annihilation
The process of producing a positron and a negatron that are each equal to 0.51

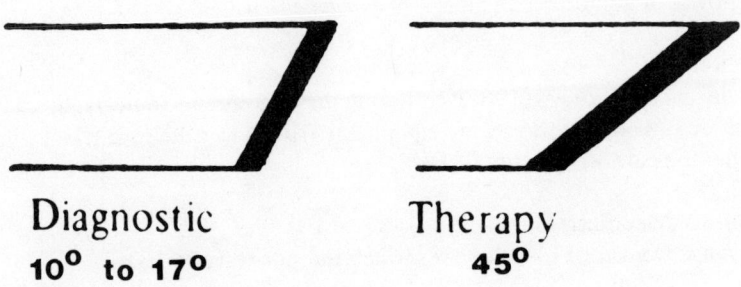

Angulation of Anode

mev. This process occurs when photon energy is at 1.02 mev during pair production. See *pair production*.

annihilation radiation
Electromagnetic radiation produced by annihilation of an positron and an electron. Each such annihilation usually produces two photons, which have the same properties as gamma rays.

anode
Positive electrode or terminal to which electrons are attracted.

anode cooling curve chart
This chart is provided with each tube to indicate the rate at which heat is dissipated in terms of minutes. The chart must be consulted before making a series of rapid exposures. See illustration.

anode thermal capacity
The quantitative ability of the anode portion of the x-ray tube to store and withstand large amounts of heat.

AOT
See *Schonander*.

aperture diaphragm
One form of a beam restrictor consisting of lead blocked designed sheet with various openings suitable to cover a given size film at a given distance.

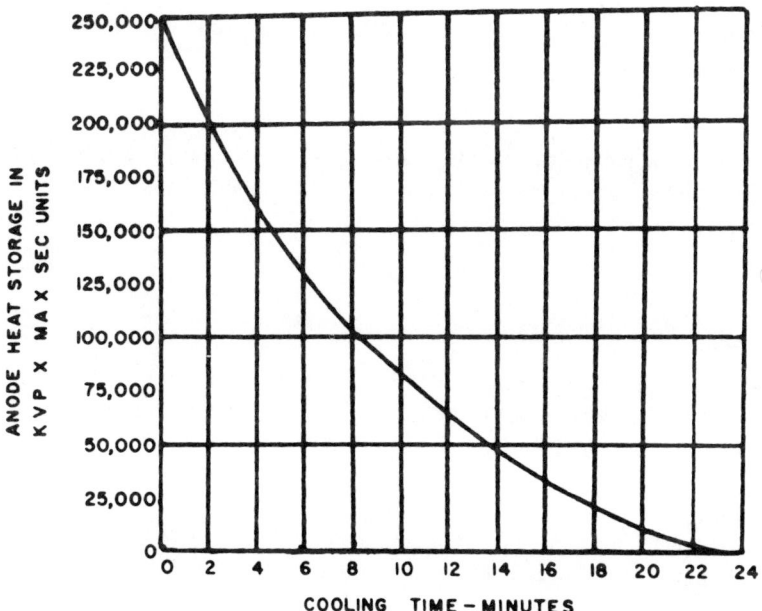

Anode Cooling Curve Chart

apron (lead protective)
During fluoroscopy, the radiologists and the technologists are required to wear lead rubber aprons of .5mm lead equivalent.

archival storage, CT
Long term storage of information. In CT this can be accomplished by storing the information on digital magnetic tape, floppy disk, or as images on x-ray film.

arcing
Sparking effect that may occur between the cathode and anode, caused by a malfunction.

armature
The part of a generator or motor that rotates between the field poles and carrying windings in which the electromotive force acts for operating the machine.

armature coil
A coil of wire placed on the armature of a generator or motor; part of the armature winding.

armature core
The core cylinder or ring on which, or in which, armature windings are carried.

artifact (artefact)
A mark on the x-ray film due to an accident or rough handling during the processing.

artifact, CT
An error in the reconstructed image that has no counterpart in reality. It may be produced by a machine peculiarity, by the mathematics of the reconstruction, or by an error of the operator.

artificial permanent magnet
See *hard steel* and *alnico*.

artificial radioactive isotopes
Bombarding the element with protons, neutrons, gamma rays or other particles under controlled conditions as in a cyclotron or reactor.

ASA rating
Speed rating of photographic materials devised by the American Standards Association. The rating is based on an arithmetical progression using an average gradient system.

A scan
A misnomer for A mode or for scanning with A mode display.

atom
The smallest particle of an element that has the characteristics of that element and can combine chemically with one or more atoms of another element. There are 103 known kinds of atoms, each having a different arrangement of electrons and protons. See illustration.

atomic
Pertaining to atoms.

atomic mass
The number of protons and neutrons in the nucleus of an atom. Also called *atomic weight* or *nucleic mass*. Formerly called *isotopic mass*.

atomic mass unit (amu)
A unit of mass equal to one-sixteenth the mass of oxygen.

atomic nucleus
The central area of the atom, made up of the protons and neutrons.

atomic number
Symbol Z. The number of protons in the nucleus of an atom. It is a different

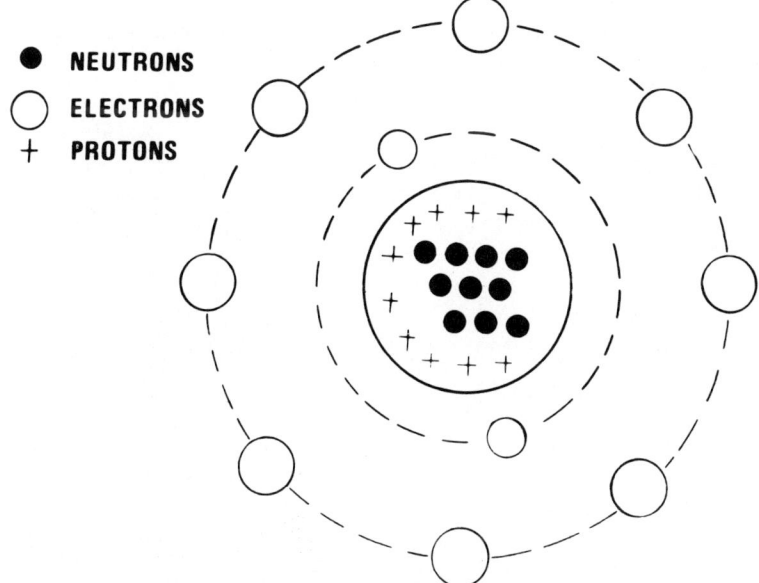

Atom

number for each element. For a neutral atom, the number is also the number of electrons outside the nucleus.

atomic orbit
The uniform circles outside of the nucleus that carry the electron of a given atom.

atomic shell
Lettered orbital path of an atom.

atomic theory
The concept that an atom consists of a central positively charged nucleus having considerable mass or weight and surrounded by a number of electrons moving in orbits at a relatively great distance from the nucleus.

atomic weight
Number of protons and neutrons in an atom. Can also be referred to as *atomic mass* or *mass number*.

attenuation
When radiation passes through matter, this radiation loses energy, and this is said to be attenuation of radiation.

attenuation coefficient
The ratio of change of x-ray beam strength (photons) through a material in comparison to a prescribed attenuation standard. See *linear attenuation coefficient*.

attenuator
A control device consisting of a network of circuit units, such as resistors, capacitors, and conductors designed to decrease the signal strength by a controlled amount.

automatic collimation
Process by which the collimator automatically adjusts to the size of the cassette when placed in the Bucky tray.

automatic exposure control
Circuits integrated into the x-ray system that automatically terminate the exposure when the desired densities on a film are produced.

automatic line voltage compensator
Automatic electronic control of the incoming power supply. It guarantees ± 10 percent of the factors density selected at the control panel. Superior to the standard manual line voltage compensator.

automatic pressure injector
Machine used for special procedure examinations requiring rapid injection of contrast material, for example, angiography.

automatic processing
A film processing unit in which developing, fixing, washing, and drying of a film is accomplished mechanically. There are many units on the market, for example, *X-omats*. See illustration.

automatic serial changer
Machine used generally in special procedures for rapid filming of examinations, for example, *angiography*.

autoradiography
Record of radiation from radioactive material in an object made by placing the object in close proximity to a photographic emulsion.

autotomography
Tomography obtained by the patient slowly moving his/her head during exposure. Primary use was in pneumoencephalography or angiography.

autotransformer
A single coil transformer that can step-up or step-down voltages. It varies the

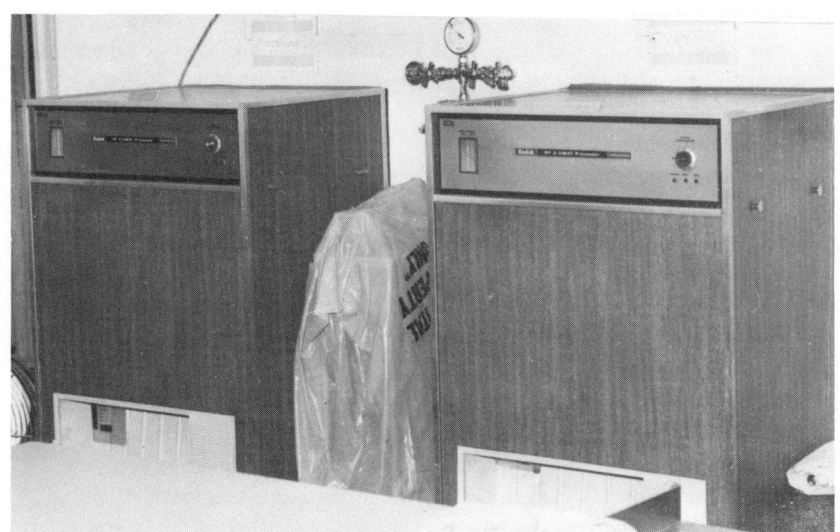

Automatic Processing

voltage input to the primary of the high voltage transformer. This transformer is self-inducted coil and serves as a Kv. selector.

average deviation
See *mean deviation*.

average gradient
The measurement of the scope or steepness of the straight line of the H & D curve between 0.25 and 2.00.

average life
See *half-life*.

Avogadro's number
Number of atoms in a gram atomic weight of any element. Also the number of molecules in the gram molecular weight of any substance.

axial, CT
The circular movement of the x-ray source around the patient to provide multi-directional x-ray transmission to a detector system.

axial (depth) resolution
The ability to distinguish two objects on a line parallel to the sound source. Measured as a distance between objects when they are just resolvable.

back emf
Electromotive force that backs up during self-induction and opposes the applied electromotive force; this is called bucking.

background radiation
The radiation of man's natural environment, including that which comes from cosmic rays, from the naturally radioactive elements of the earth, and from within man's body.

backscatter
Radiation deflected back through the plane of entry into an object.

ballistic milliampere–second meter
In x-ray equipment operating at 200 mA. or more, this meter is necessary to register the mA.S. at a slower swing of the needle so that it can be easily read with exposures below 1/10 second. This meter measures tube current and must be used in conjunction with the impulse and electronic timers. With any exposure above 1/10 second, the ordinary milliammeter will register the correct milliamperage.

bandwidth
The total number of cycles per unit of time (usually one second) that may be used to modulate the electron beam in a television camera.

bank resistors
See *space charge compensator.*

barium
Symbol *Ba*, is used for testing abnormalities of the gastrointestinal tract.

barium fluorochloride
A fluorescent material used in the manufacture of intensifying screens.

barium lead sulfate
A fluorescent material used in the manufacture of intensifying screens.

barium platinocyanide
Used in the manufacturing of intensifying screens. The chemical substance used in the discovery of x-ray by Dr. W. C. Roentgen.

barium strontium sulfate
A fluorescent material used in the manufacture of intensifying screens.

barium sulfate
The term barium is usually used to refer to barium sulfate, an insoluble com-

pound of barium and sulfuric acid, that is used as a contrast medium in medical radiography because of its high radiopacity.

base, x-ray film
A transparent sheet of polyester plastic material of about 0.2mm (8 mils or 0.008 in.) thickness that is usually tinted blue violet or green sensitive. The base holds the emulsion of silver bromide crystal on both sides.

base density
See *base fog.*

base fog
Density on x-ray film that is below 0.25 on the H & D curve. Also called *base density.*

battery
A d.c. voltage supply made up of one or more cells to change chemical, nuclear, thermal, or solar energy into electrical energy.

beam
See *x-ray beam.*

beam barrier (diagnostic)
According to the appropriate table in Handbook 76, the average diagnostic tube requires a 1.5 mm (1/16 inch) lead.

beam flattening filter
Special filter used in betatrons and linear accelerators, for x-ray beams, to obtain flat isodose curves.

beam restrictor
Metallic devices that are attached to the x-ray tube housing to limit the beam to the field of interest. They are: aperture diaphragms, cones and collimators. See illustration.

beamsplitter
An optical element used to divide a beam of light so that it may be projected simultaneously in two different directions.

bedside radiography
X-ray examination taken at the patient's bed with a portable x-ray unit.

beryllium window
The windows of the x-ray tubes are generally constructed of beryllium.

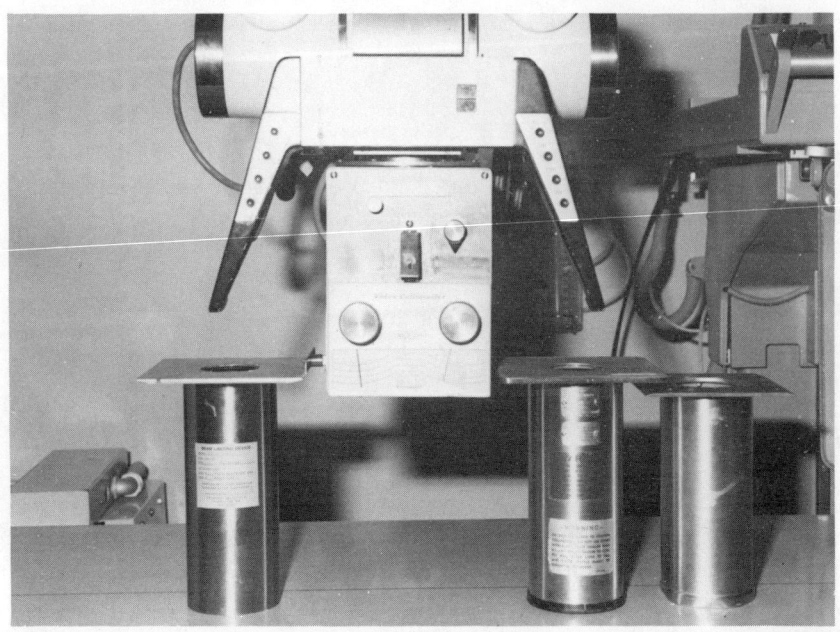

Beam Restrictor

beta decay
Radioactive transformation of a nuclide in which the atomic number increases or decreases by one and the mass number remains unchanged. The atomic number increases when a negative beta particle (negatron) is emitted and decreases when a positive beta-particle (positron) is emitted or an electron is captured.

beta particles
High speed electrons that penetrate matter to a greater depth than alpha rays. They are used in therapy for superficial skin lesions.

beta rays
Electrons emitted by radioactive particles. See *beta particles*.

betatron
A magnetic induction accelerator that makes use of a varying magnetic field to accelerate electrons. Electrons are injected into a toroidal vacuum chamber which is between the poles of an iron-core magnet. The rate of change of the magnet flux and magnetic field at the orbit radius are related to maintain a constant radius for the accelerating electrons.

bias
See *grid, electronic.*

binding energy (atomic)
That energy which holds the electron to its given shell. The binding energy of the K shell is the largest because the K electron is closest to the nucleus.

binocular stereoscope
The simplest type of a hand-held portable stereoscopic unit, having two 20° prisms, one being held before each eye.

biological effect (radiation)
The result that radiation may have on life and living organisms in general.

biological half-life
The time required for radioactivity in an organism to diminish to half its original value by natural biological excretion processes.

biophysics
The science which deals with the physical processes of living tissues and organisms.

bi-plane
In special procedures, the process of taking films in two planes utilizing a single injection of contrast media.

bit CT
The smallest unit of digital information expressed in the binary system of notation (either a 0 or a 1).

bite-wing
A dental film placed between the occlusal surface of the teeth for the survey of teeth bite.

black level
That level in the composite video signal at which the kinescope electron beam is completely extinguished.

blanking
That period of time during the television scanning process when the electron beam is automatically driven to the blank level for retrace.

blood count
Blood counts should be done periodically for radiation workers for early detec-

tion of radiation injury. However, it is not a substitute for film badges and other monitoring devices.

blooming focal spot
A focal spot may become larger (bloom) with an increase of mA, however, it will decrease in size with an increase in Kv.P. It is important to realize that in angiography, for example, the focal spot increases about 50 percent when going from 200 to 1000 mA.

B mode
Brightness modulation. Echoes displayed as illuminated dots along a baseline—represent time. Brightness proportional to the amplitude of the echo.

body (human) atomic number
See *effective atomic number.*

body section radiography (tomography)
A special x-ray apparatus that layers thin body sections at any predetermined depth in focus and blurs out the body sections above and below this predetermined section. Body section radiography is known as tomography and is variously described as planigraphy, laminagraphy, stratigraphy, ordography, and otherwise according to manufacturer.

Bohr Theory
That the atom represented a miniature solar system analogue to the sun with planets revolving about it. Niels Bohr, 1913.

boiling off electrons
Heat or incandescense of the filament of the x-ray tube for a source of electrons. See *thermionic emission* (effect).

bolus
A volume of injected tracer or x-ray contrast medium that travels in the body without substantial dispersion during a study.

bone age radiograph
A multiview series of x-ray to determine the maturation or growth of bones compared with tabulated standards.

bone radiation absorption
The effective atomic number of bone is 11.6, which will absorb more radiation than fat, muscle, or water.

booster circuit
Part of the filament circuit that will raise the filament current to the peak selected value just before the exposure is to be made.

bound electron
An electron that is close to the nucleus, for example, the K shell electron.

brachytherapy
Therapy at short distances with beta or gamma radiation. Implantation or placement therapy with needles, inserts, or other such applications containing radioactive materials.

"break"
Referring to the instant the switch is opened or electrical switch is turned off.

B ray
Emitted from the nucleus during beta decay.

Bremsstrahlung Radiation
That radiation produced when fastmoving negative electrons strike a positive anode of an x-ray tube. Frequently called brems or braking radiation.

bridge circuit
A circuit consisting basically of four valve tubes connected in series to form a diamond. The a.c. source is then changed to a d.c. after passing through the bridge circuit. This system is more commonly called full-wave rectification. See *full-wave rectification.*

brightness control
A potentiometer (varies voltages) connected in the television circuit, that controls the brightness of screen image. Also called *brilliance control* and *intensity control.*

British Thermal Unit (B.T.U.)
The quantity of heat required to increase the temperature of one pound of water one degree Fahrenheit at atmospheric pressure; approximately 252 gram-calories.

brushes
Conductive metal rings at the end of the armature of a generator connecting to the external circuit for the purpose of withdrawing the current.

bucks
Opposition of the applied emf to the source of power (generator or battery) during self-induction coils.

Bucky diaphragm
In 1909, Dr. Gustave Bucky invented a radiographic apparatus consisting of a grid of parallel lead strips with radiolucent materials between the lead strips.

The primary purpose is to clean up secondary radiation and to enhance radiographic contrast

Bucky table
An x-ray table having a Bucky tray and a grid.

Bucky tray
Found beneath the x-ray table and grid. This tray, which slides in and out, is used to hold the cassette during the exposure.

Bucky wallstand
A cassette holder apparatus fastened to the wall in a vertical position. Usually called *wallstand cassette holder.*

Bunsen-Roscoe
See *reciprocity law.*

cable
Conductive wires connected from the x-ray transformer to the x-ray tube. They are shockproof and insulated to prevent sparking.

cadmium
Symbol *Cd.* A metallic element of importance as a control absorber and shield in nuclear reactors.

cadmium zinc sulfide
See *zinc cadmium sulfide.*

calcium tungstate
A fluorescent material used in the manufacture of intensifying screens.

calibrate
To determine, by measurement, the settings of a control that correspond to particular values of voltage, current, frequency, or some other electrical characteristics of an x-ray machine.

calibration
Determination of variation from standard, or accuracy, of a measuring instrument to ascertain necessary correction factors.

caliper
A tool to measure thickness of the body parts.

Camp's grid cassette
A cassette having a thin wafer grid on the front part of the cassette. Invented by Dr. John D. Camp.

capacitance
Symbol C. A quantity of electricity in coulombs stored per volt applied to the capacitor. The unit of measurement is a farad.

capacitive reactance
The resistance to the flow of an a.c. current by a capacitor.

capacitor
Symbol *C*. A device consisting essentially of two conducting surfaces separated by a dielectric material such as air, paper, mica, ceramic, or glass. A capacitor stores electric energy, blocks direct current, and permits alternating current to flow. Also called a *condenser*. See illustration.

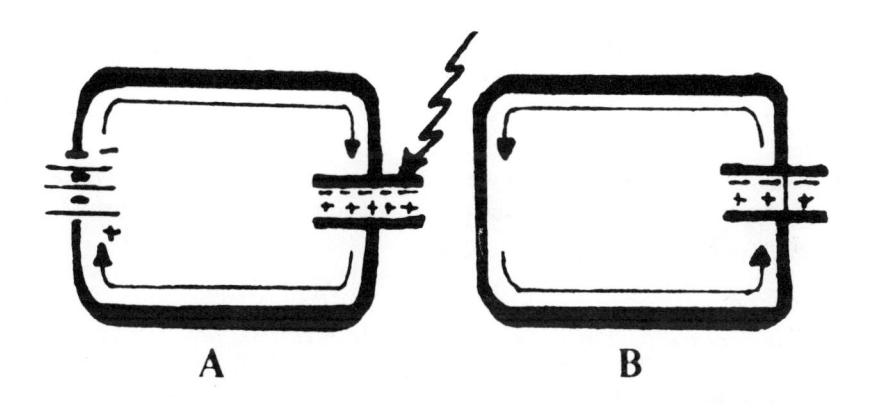

Capacitor   "A" plate is being negatively charged and "B" plate is being positively charged.

capacity
The extent to which a capacitor or condenser can be charged with electrical energy.

carbon
An element widely used in the construction of resistors, dry cells, and nuclear reactors.

carbon-fibre
Low absorption material used on compression plates of Schonander and Puck-cut film changers to reduce radiation and improve the radiographic image.

cardboard film holder
A light-tight film container made of heavy cardboard and paper, used in radiography.

C-arm
See *mobile intensifier.*

cassette (radiographic)
An x-ray film holder containing intensifying screens mounted within front and back structures which are hinged together. The x-ray film is placed between the intensifying screens to prepare the cassette for use.

cassette changer
A piece of radiographic equipment designed for quick changing of cassettes so that successive exposures may be made without changing the position of the patient, as in stereoscopy.

cassette tunnel
A tunnel apparatus designed so that a cassette can be placed beneath the tunnel and removed without moving the tunnel. Useful for O.R. hip pinnings.

catalyst
A substance that alters the velocity of a chemical reaction without undergoing any apparent physical or chemical change itself and without becoming a part of the product formed.

cathode
Negative electrode or terminal that gives off electrons.

cathode cable
The cable for the cathode terminal has three contacts that lead to the two filaments of a double focus tube and one that leads to the secondary side of the high voltage transformer.

cathode rays
The stream of electrons that travel from cathode to anode in an x-ray or valve tube. Measured in milliamperes by the milliammeter placed in the high voltage circuit. More technically called *tube current.*

cathode ray tube, CT
The abbreviation crt refers to the television-type screen presentation used to display processed scans (for diagnosis and photography) and/or alphanumeric information. Used synonymously with *vdu* (*video display unit.*)

cation
A positive ion which flows to the cathode of an electric solution (cell) and gives up a positive charge.

catphantom
This phantom is designed to be used in checking all CT system image parameters

across the entire spectrum of CT numbers. It is designed to minimize CT system time required for Quality Assurance Programs. The modular construction of this tool encourages the insertion sections for dosimetry, in vitro specimen studies, and other research needs.

cell
A single unit of a battery that generates chemical energy into electrical energy.

celsius
See *centigrade*.

centi- (c)
A prefix representing 10^{-2}, which is 0.01 or one-hundredth.

centigrade (C)
The metric temperature scale on which the freezing point of water is 0° and the boiling point of water is 100°. Formula for conversion of centigrade to Fahrenheit:

$$F = \frac{9}{5}C + 32$$

centimeter (cm)
A unit of length in the metric system, equal to 0.01 meter or 0.394 in. 2.54 cm = 1 in.

centimeter-gram-second
Metric system meaning centimeter-length, gram-mass, and second-time.

central beam
See *central ray*.

central ray
The theoretical center of the x-ray beam. The central ray leaves the focal spot at 90° from the long axis of the tube housing. Also called *central beam*.

centrifugal force
A force that tends to impel a thing or parts of a thing outward from a center of rotation.

centripetal force
A force proceeding or acting in a direction toward the center axis.

Certificate of Need
Governmental program initiated to regulate major capital expenditures and changes in service of health care facilities.

cesium
Used in radiotherapy for therapy at intermediate depths.

"chalky" radiograph
A film with excessive high contrast, images too white, lacing gray tones.

chamber, ionization
See *ionization chamber* and *Victoreen R-meter*.

changeover switch
An electrical switch that permits the fluorographer to switch from fluoroscopy to spot film work automatically.

changer
See *automatic serial changer*.

characteristic curve
A curve that is plotted with the logarithm of exposure on a horizontal scale and optical density, which is a logarithmic measurement vertically.

characteristic radiation
Radiation originating in an atom following removal of an electron. The wavelength of the emitted radiation depends only on the element concerned and the energy levels involved. When an electron of an atom moves from a higher level of electron energy, the energy given off in this movement is called characteristic radiation.

characteristic x-rays
See *characteristic radiation*.

charge
The amount (quantity) of electricity.

chemical behavior (properties)
The ability of the element to unite with another is dependent upon the valence of the element.

chemical bond
An attraction between two ions. Also called *ionic polar valence*.

chemical energy
See *battery* or *cell*.

chemical fog
Fogging due to developing at excessively high temperatures or overdevelopment;

oxidized, deteriorated developer; prolonged or repeated inspection of films during development; and contaminated tanks.

choke coil
Variable resistor working on the electromagnetic self-induction principle, using alternating current only.

cine camera
A camera used for recording motion (in cinefluoroscopy one which usually utilizes either 16 or 35 mm film). Frame rates may be on the order of 15 to 60 frames per second.

cine fluoroscopy
Procedure used to make motion pictures directly from the output phosphor of the image intensifier.

cineradiography
See *cine fluoroscopy*.

circuit
An arrangement of one or more complete paths for electron flow. A circuit consists of three main parts: potential difference, current strength, and resistance.

circuit booster
Is found in the filament circuit to limit the filament current at a low value until the x-ray exposure switch is closed. The apparatus is called a booster.

circuit breaker
An electromagnetic device that terminates the exposure automatically when the current exceeds a predetermined value.

circuit diagram, x-ray
See schematic diagram on p. 187.

clearing time
The amount of fixer time it requires to remove all the unexposed silver salts from a film.

closed circuit
A complete path for current to travel.

closed core transformer
The primary and secondary coils which are highly insulated from each other are wrapped around a square connected type of core. Commonly called the *doughnut transformer*.

cloud electron
See *thermionic emission*.

coaxial cable
A type of special cable used to transmit the composite video signal from the camera to the monitor and/or magnetic recorders. The signal conductor, in the center of the cable, has a protective grounded metallic sheath around it.

cobalt
Symbol *Co*. A metallic element combined with iron and steel to make special alloys used in permanent magnets.

cobalt 60
A radioisotope having a half-life of 5.3 years.

coherent scattering
Sometimes called unmodified scattering. One of the four interactions that occur when photons (x-rays) and atoms collide with each other. The low energy x-ray photon collides with a inner-orbital electron, but its low energy cannot dislodge the electron. The electron may absorb the photon which then will set the photon into vibration causing an electromagnetic wave, the same as the incident (incoming) photon, but in a different direction. This type of interaction is below the energy range useful in clinical radiology.

cohesion
A force that unites the particles of a body.

coil
Symbol L. A copper wire wound in a bedspring-shaped helix around a soft iron core for the purpose of building a magnetic inductance as used for transformers and other electrical devices.

cold area
Radiosotopic scanning area where no activity is registered. This is usually an indication of an abnormality.

collimation
The process of confining the radiation to the field of interest.

collimator
One form of a beam restrictor which is a box-like apparatus with two sets of adjustable diaphragms placed one above the other corresponding to the upper and lower apertures of a cone that can be opened or closed to any desired rectangular size.

collision
A close approach of two or more objects (particles, photons, atomic or nuclear systems) during which there occurs an interchange of quantities such as energy, momentum, and charge.

colloid
A substance that disperses particles in a medium. The gelatin of the film emulsion could be called a colloid.

commutator
An electrical device designed to reverse the flow of electrical current. Placed at the end of the armature of a d.c. generator, it takes out current to the external circuit which travels in one direction only.

commutator ring
See *commutator*.

compass
The simplest device for detection of magnetism. It is made up of a north magnetic needle that points to the earth's north pole. So that the compass north needle points to the north pole, it is made up of a south magnetic material.

compensating filters
Filtering devices adding radiographic density for the parts of the body that differ greatly in thickness, so that these areas can be of even densities on a given radiograph. The thickest part of the aluminum wedge is placed at the thinnest part of the body.

compensator
See *line voltage compensator*.

complex pattern, ultrasound
Any structure that is recorded which gives the appearance of having both solid and cystic components.

composite video signal
The complete television signal transmitted from the camera; it consists of three parts: video, blanking, and synchronizing pulses.

compound
Complex substances formed by the chemical union of two or more elements.

compound molecule
Is a substance that contains atoms of more than one kind.

compound scanning, ultrasound
Also known as *sectoring*. Applies to the way in which the transducer is moved across the patient involving a series of arcing motions of the transducer often moving the transducer over the same area many times to "build up" an image.

compression cone
This device is an attachment for use in fluoroscopy of the GI tract and serves to permit the examiner to apply pressure to various parts being examined, displace some of the overlying structures, and improve the radiographic examination.

compression device
A mechanical means for reducing the thickness of a part of the body for the purpose of improving the radiographic examination. One type is used for IVP work (primarily for compression of the ureters) and other types are used in fluoroscopy of the GI tract.

compression technique
A radiographic examination using pressure or pressure devices to limit contrast media to a particular area of interest.

Compton effect
See *Compton scatter radiation*.

Compton scatter radiation
Commonly called scatter radiation. That radiation having sufficient energy to dislodge a bound electron, but attacks a loosely bound electron, dislodges the electron and this energy proceeds in a different direction. See illustration.

computer assisted tomography
See *computerized tomography*.

computerized tomography (CT)
The technique by which multidirectional x-ray transmission data through a body is mathematically reconstructed by a computer to form an electrical cross-sectional representation (slice) of a patient's anatomy. CT is used as an acronym to designate any technical field associated with these techniques.

condenser
See *capacitor*.

conductance
A measure of the ability of a material to conduct electric current. It is the reciprocal of the resistance of the material, and is expressed in ohms.

conductivity
See *conductance*.

PHOTON (X-RAY)

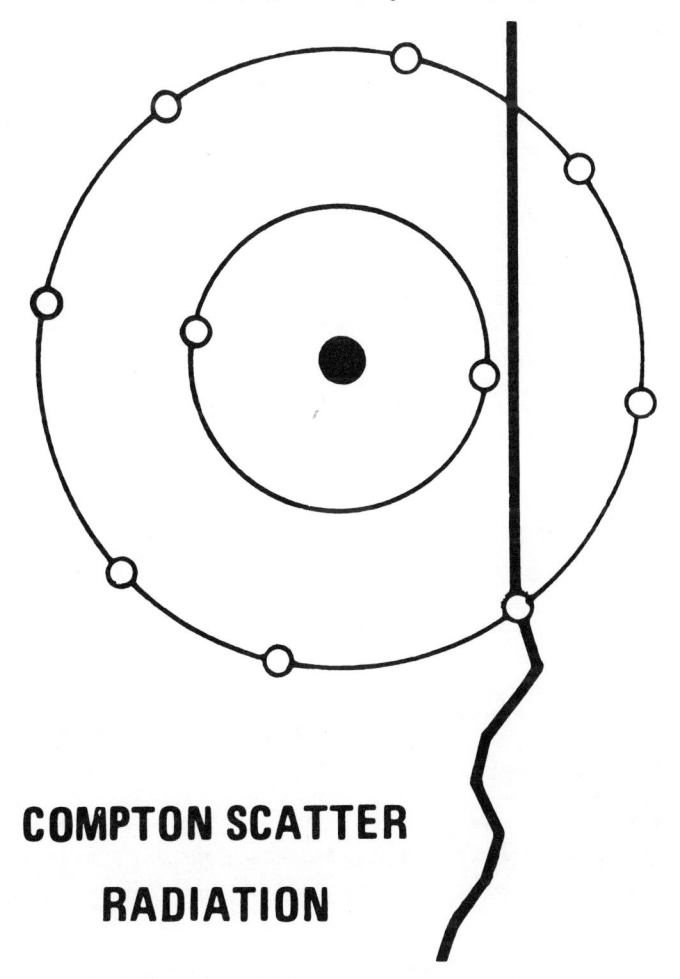

COMPTON SCATTER RADIATION

Compton Scatter Radiation

conductor
Material, usually metal, having low electrical resistance that will allow electricity to flow freely, for example, silver or copper. A conductor's atom valence structure is loose, meaning that electrons may flow freely.

cone
A metallic circular device that is attached to the x-ray tube housing to limit the beam to the field of interest.

connection
The place of union between two electrical points allowing electricity to flow.

connector
An electrical device to connect two points, for example, a mating plug or receptacle.

constant potential
Term applied to unidirectional potential (one direction voltage) that has little or no magnitude of ripple of the sine wave.

constant-potential circuit
This particular circuit has been fully rectified, but because of the space that exists between each alternation, a charged capacitor ripples energy from peak to peak.

contact (electrical)
A conducting part of a relay, connector, or switch that will unite with another such part to make or break the electrical flow of a circuit.

contrast media (agent)
A substance substantially different in density from the surrounding structures so that when instilled within the body, the internal structures can be outlined for the purpose of radiography.

contrast, radiographic
The visible differentiation between bony structure and tissue opacity as indicated by the degrees of gray tones. See *long (low) scale contrast* and *short scale contrast*.

control grid
A grid, ordinarily placed between the cathode and the anode, serves to control the anode current of an electron tube. See *triode tube*.

control panel
An area off of each radiographic room having a lead wall enclosure around the control board. The operator stands behind the lead wall enclosure to make the necessary factor changes and x-ray exposure.

conventional theory of current
This theory, still used by the older electricians, claims that current flows from the positive terminal through the circuit to the negative terminal. This conventional theory, which was used until 1950, has been changed to the electron theory. See *electron theory*.

convergence lines
They are imaginary lines extending from the focal spot of the x-ray tube to

the lead strips of a focused grid. The lines slant from the point at the focal spot outward to the angle of the lead strips of the focused grid.

converter
See *rotary converter*.

Coolidge transformer
Referring to the step-down transformer of the filament circuit.

Coolidge tube
The hot cathode x-ray tube designed by Wm. D. Coolidge in 1913, having a hot filament source of electrons, a tungsten target anode, and placed in a vacuum glass envelope. The same principles of basic construction of this tube obtain in the modern x-ray tubes.

copper
Symbol *Cu*. A metallic element having good electrical conductivity. Atomic number is 29. See *conductor*.

copper loss
One of the electrical power losses of transformers due to the large-sized copper conductor windings.

core iron
A grade of soft iron suitable for cores of chokes, transformers, and relays. See *soft iron*.

corner cutter
See *film corner cutter*.

corpuscular radiation (emission)
Electromagnetic radiation consisting of a shower of particles such as electrons, protons, neutrons, and others traveling at the speed of light and having no electrical charge.

cosmic rays
Highly penetrating radiation originating outside the atmosphere of the earth. Also called *background radiation*.

coulomb
Smallest part of current, named for the French physicist, C. A. Coulomb.

counter electromotive force
See *back emf*.

coupling
Mutual point between two electrical circuits where electricity can pass while the switch is closed.

coupling agent, ultrasound
Commonly used coupling agent is mineral oil. Some type of coupling agent must be used when producing a sonogram since it is critical that there be no air gaps or bubbles between the face of the transducer and the patient's skin. Therefore, a coupling agent is applied to the patient's skin and the transducer is able to glide across the area to be scanned.

crest voltmeter
A voltmeter reading the peak or maximum value of the voltage applied to its terminal.

crinkle mark
A curved black or white line which results from bending the film over the end of a finger or fingernail.

Crookes Tube
A vacuum discharge tube used by Dr. Roentgen in the discovery of x-ray. Used by Sir William Crookes in early experimental works.

crosshatch grid
Two stationary grids, one having lead strips running at the long axis, and the second grid having lead strips running at right angles to the first one. Not used for routine radiography; may be used for special radiographic examination.

crystal
Referring to intensifying screen, the size of the crystals determines the speed of the screen; for example, the smaller the screen's crystals, the slower the screen, but the greater the radiographic definition.

CT numbers
The numbers used to designate the x-ray attentuation in each picture element of the CT image.

cubic centimeter
Equal to 1/1000 liter.

cumulative dose (radiation)
The total dose resulting from repeated exposures to radiation.

curie
Unit of radioactive material 3.700×10^{10} nuclear transformations per second.

Curie, Marie
The Polish chemist who discovered radium and polonium in 1898; her husband, Pierre, was the codiscoverer.

current
Symbol I. Unit of an ampere, electron in motion.

current stabilizer
A device that functions so that considerable changes in the voltages are accompanied by relatively little change in the filament current. This maintenance of nearly constant filament current results from use of a condenser and small transformer in the primary circuit.

cutie pie
A portable ionization chamber survey meter.

cycle
Complete sequence of alternating current having positive and negative alternations. Sixty cycle a.c. is used in the incoming lines of x-ray units in the United States. See illustration.

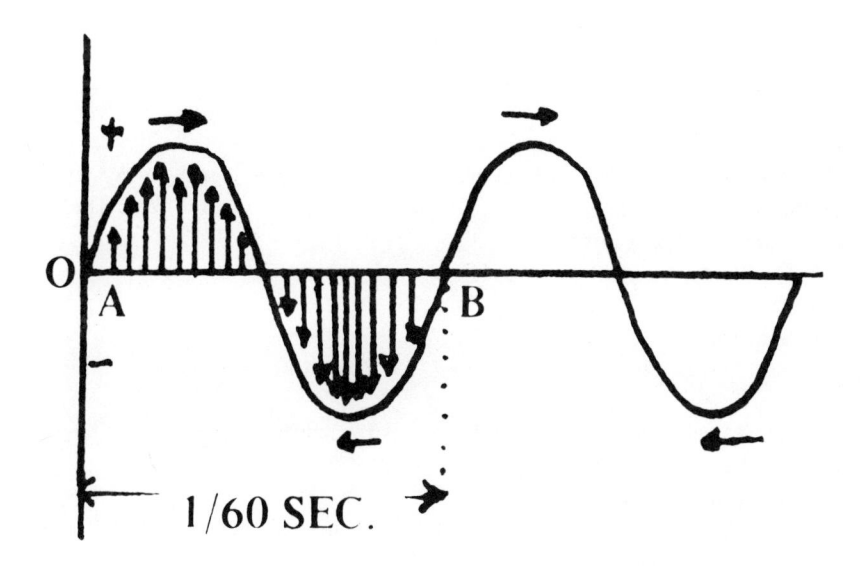

Cycle

cycles per second (cps)
Unit of frequency. Also called hertz. Sixty cycle a.c. is used in the United States for incoming electrical lines.

cyclotron
An accelerator used to produce high energy protons, deuterons, and other relatively heavy charged particles. Energies of the order of 20 MEV to 100 MEV may be achieved in modified versions. Such particles may be used for basic physics research. They are sometimes used medically directly for experimental therapy, but more often to produce radio-nuclides and neutron beams.

cycon
See *sodium sulfite*.

cylinder
A cylindrically shaped device which is sometimes used in the place of a cone. A cylinder which may be extended is called an extension cylinder.

cystic pattern
Any structure recorded which gives the appearance of being echo free. This is one of the most important patterns to recognize when scanning.

dampening
Process by which the pulse duration is shortened.

darkroom
A lightproof room adequately ventilated for the purposes of handling and processing x-ray film.

data acquisition system (DAS)
The components of a CT machine used to produce and collect the x-ray attenuation information: x-ray tube, detectors, and detector preamplifiers. These are mounted on the gantry.

daughter
Synonym for *decay product*.

data
Term used for numbers, letters, and symbols for record keeping.

daylight system
Method of loading, unloading, and feeding films into the processor in normal room light. This system entails the use of special equipment and there is no need for a darkroom. See illustration.

d.c. generator
Direct current generator is a mechanical device to produce a d.c. power supply by rotating the armature so that the commutator ring supplies the external circuit with pulsating direct current.

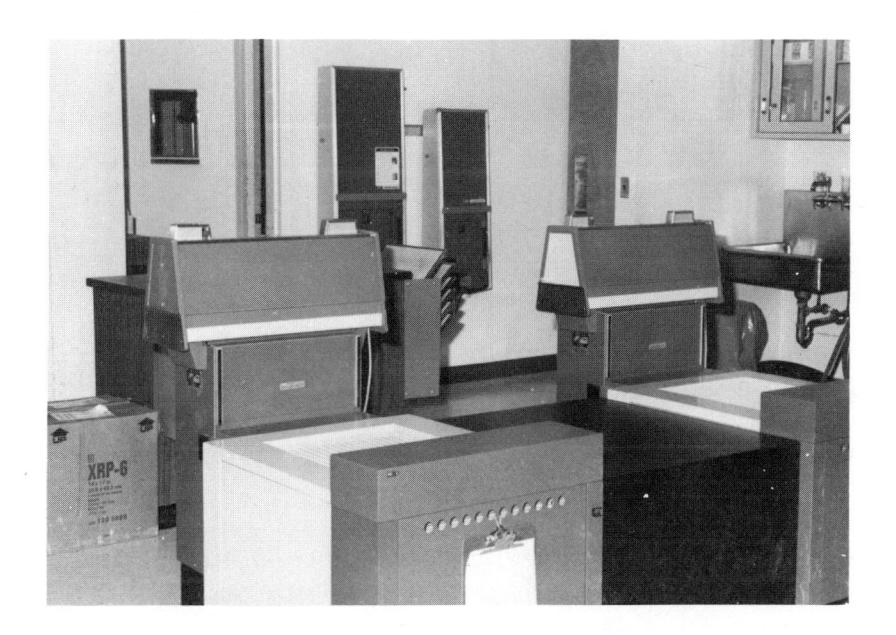

Daylight System

dead man switch
A switch so constructed that a circuit-closing contact can be maintained only by continuous pressure on the switch.

dead time
An interval or recovery time of a G-M and a scintillation counter following a pulse. A correction factor of a scintillation counter is 1 percent, and of a G-M counter, 11 percent.

decay product
A nuclide resulting from the radioactive disintegration of radionuclides. Decay products may be either stable or radioactive.

decay, radioactive
Gradual reduction of strength of a radiation source.

decibel (db)
A means of expressing the ratio of two intensities. For voltage, as would be the case with a television signal, it equals 20 times the logarithm (to the base 10) of the ratio of the two intensities.

deep therapy
A term used in radiation therapy when the effects of treatment are maximized at some depth within the tissues while sparing the skin and superficial tissues.

definition, radiographic
A diagnostic radiograph having sufficient penetration, adequate density, and visible detail sharpness.

degassing
Process of driving out gas particles occupying an electron tube (x-ray), by a heating process.

delay
Amount of time by which an electrical signal is retarded.

delay circuit
Circuit in which the output signal is delayed by a specified time interval with respect to the input signal.

delta ray
Any secondary ionizing particle ejected by recoil when a primary ionizing particle passes through matter.

delta winding
The configuration of the primary and one of the secondary coils for three-phase x-ray generators. There are two secondary coils and the star configuration is used for the other secondary coil.

demagnetization
Removal of magnetic attraction.

densitometer
Instrument used to measure the optical density of a given radiography.

density
Mass per unit volume.

density equalization filter
A radiographic accessory device that is used when it is desirable to cause a variation of x-ray intensity across a part of varying thickness.

density, radiographic
Radiographic density is the overall darkness of a radiograph.

depth dose
The depth dose is the dose of radiation delivered within the tissues at the point of interest. Among the factors important in the estimation of depth dose are: estimation of the depth of tissue of interest, kilovoltage, filtration, and size of the field. Generally measured in rad (radiation absorb dose).

depth dose data—terms
Central ray: The straight line passing through the center of the source and the center of the final beam-limiting diaphragm.

Central ray depth dose tables: Tables providing both percent depth dose and backscatter data along the central ray for various field size, beam quality, and SSD value.

depth of focus
The allowable out-of-focus condition in the image plane which may be tolerated and still maintain a specified resolving power.

detail, radiographic
The overall sharpness that is radiographically demonstrated and affected by motion, screen-film contact, focal spot size, screen unsharpness and geometric unsharpness—affecting this is the "visibility of detail."

detector
A device used to sense the occurrence of an event.

developer solution, x-ray
The purpose of the solution is to activate the exposed areas and to retard development of the unexposed areas of the film emulsion. The reducing agents are hydroquinone and metol; preservative is sodium sulfite; accelerator is sodium carbonate or sodium hydroxide; and restrainer is potassium bromide.

development, x-ray film
The function is to convert the latent image to a visible image by means of developer solution.

Diagnost 120—Philips
Remote control radiographic and fluoroscopic system.

diagnostic radiograph
A radiograph with sufficient penetration (Kv.P.), adequate density (mA.S.), and visible detail.

diamagnetic
A material that repels magnetism, for example, beryllium or bismuth.

diaphragm
See *aperture diaphragm*.

diaphragm, Bucky
See *Potter-Bucky diaphragm (bucky)*.

dielectric
Material that is not a good conductor or insulator. Found between the two plates of a capacitor.

dielectric hysteresis
Electric field lagging with respect to a.c. that is applied to the dielectric material of a capacitor.

dielectric loss
Heat loss in electric energy found in capacitors.

difference of potential
See *potential difference.*

diffusion
Shifting around of molecules through matter due to the higher increase of temperature.

dimmer
Electrical or electronic control to vary the intensity of light.

dimming circuit
Found in the filament circuit of the x-ray circuit. Even though the filaments are lit when the machine is not making exposures, they burn at a low, stand-by amperage and will flash up to the full brightness before and during the exposures. This process prolongs the life of the filament.

diode tube
A two-electrode electronic tube, for example, the x-ray and the rectifying (valve) tube, referring to the cathode and anode.

direct current (d.c.)
Electric current flowing in one direction only.

directory, CT
An area on the magnetic tape storage or magnetic disc in which a concise or abbreviated list of the stored information is available. In CT equipment, the directory may be requested for display on the CRT or as a hard-copy readout.

direct radiation
That radiation coming directly from the x-ray tube.

disk, CT
General term used for various types of magnetic recording disks used through-

out the system. Specific types or uses are designated by a descriptive name such as system disk or floppy disk. Also see *floppy disk*.

discharge, electrical
To remove a charge from a battery, capacitor, or other electric energy storage device.

disintegration, radioactive
The length of time required for the decay of radioactive elements. See also *half-life*.

display monitor
The TV screen used to display the CT image. A monitor is distinct from a TV set in that it normally does not include the tuner that allows you to select a particular channel. Monitors are therefore used in closed circuit applications.

distortion, radiographic
The elongation or the shortening of an image from its true shape.

distribution transformer
A source generator that reserves the kilovoltage and amperage (KVA) capacity for each x-ray room independently. Each roon has its own power source, which therefore assures that the density of each radiograph will be consistent. See illustration.

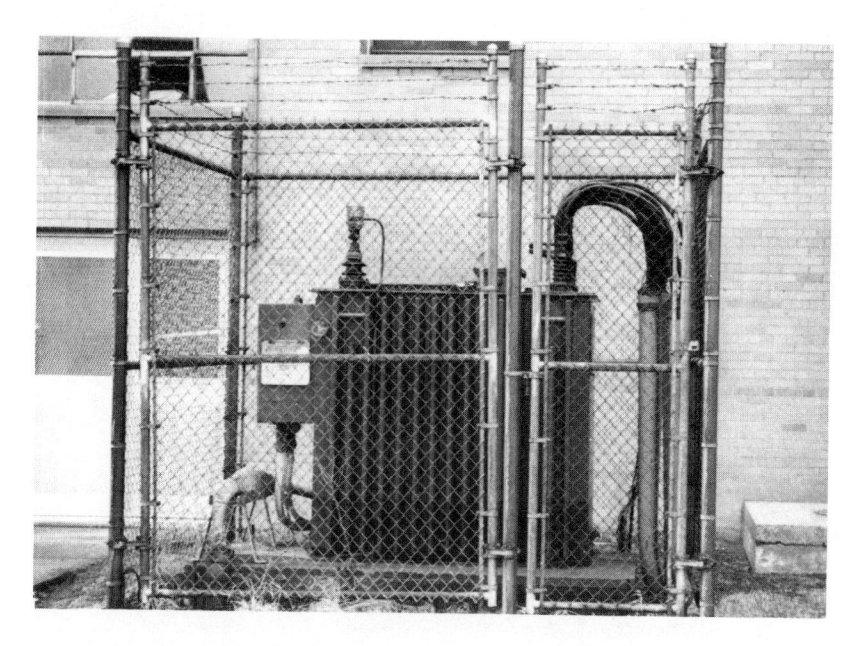

Distribution Transformer

divergence
The radiating outward from any point source of radiation.

D-Max
The abbreviation for the maximum density that a film is capable of producing. Maximum density is controlled by the amount of silver in the film's emulsion and the type of developer used during processing.

domain
See *magnetic domain*.

doppler ultrasound
A form of "continuous wave" ultrasound which measures frequency shifts. Diagnostic information is encoded as frequency shifts in returning echoes

dosage rate
The amount of radiation given per unit of time.

dose
A general form denoting the quantity of radiation or energy absorbed.

dose equivalent (DE)
The product of the absorbed dose (rad) and the appropriate modifying factors which depend on the particular radiation hazard involved.

dosimeter
An instrument for measuring doses of x-ray or of radioactivity.

dosimetry
Determination of cumulative radiation dose with radiographic or photographic film and density measurement.

double exposure
Two superimposed exposures on the same film.

double focus tube
An x-ray tube having two focal spots, one of which is smaller than the other. The smaller one is used for maximum detail, the larger one to permit greater energy to be applied to the tube.

double-pole single throw (dpst)
A four-terminal switch or relay contact arrangement that simultaneously opens or closes two separate circuits or both sides of the same circuit.

doughnut transformer
See *closed core transformer.*

drier, film
An enamel or stainless steel cabinet having racks which hold the wet films. A source of heat is usually a part of the system for rapid drying.

drop
See *voltage drop.*

dry cell
A carbon cell. The anode terminal is a carbon rod. The cathode is zinc placed in a chemical paste of sal ammoniac.

dynamo
See *generator.*

dynamo rule
See *left-hand rule.*

dyne
The unit of force which, when acting upon a mass of one gram, will produce an acceleration of one centimeter per second.

dynode
That section of a photomultiplier tube in which secondary electrons are emitted, thus providing amplification.

earth
British usage for electrical ground.

earthed
Referring to the circuit as being grounded or electrically hazardless.

eddy current
A minimal current loss due to heating of the core of a transformer. Can be reduced by using laminated silicon plates insulated from each other.

edge gradient
See *resolution.*

Edison effect
Emission of visible light, such as light from intensifying screen when struck with x-rays.

Edison's fluoroscope
A hand fluoroscope used by Thomas Edison for his experiments in 1896.

Edison, Thomas
Developed the calcium tungstate fluorescent screens that were first used by Dr. Michael Pupin of Columbia University in 1896.

effective atomic number
A number derived from the atomic numbers of a compound of mixture based on its composition. For example, the number of the human body sections, such as fat 6.3; muscle 7.4; water 7.4; and bone 11.6. Each varies in atomic number because of tissue opacity and depth of matter.

effective current
The value of alternating current that will do the same work as the corresponding value of direct current. The effective current is 0.707 times the maximum current.

effective focal spot
The perpendicular projection or effective size of the actual focal spot as it is presented to the film. The x-rays leave the rectangular actual focal spot and appear to be coming from a much smaller square area. In effect, the x-rays are emitted from the square area or the effective focal spot. See illustration.

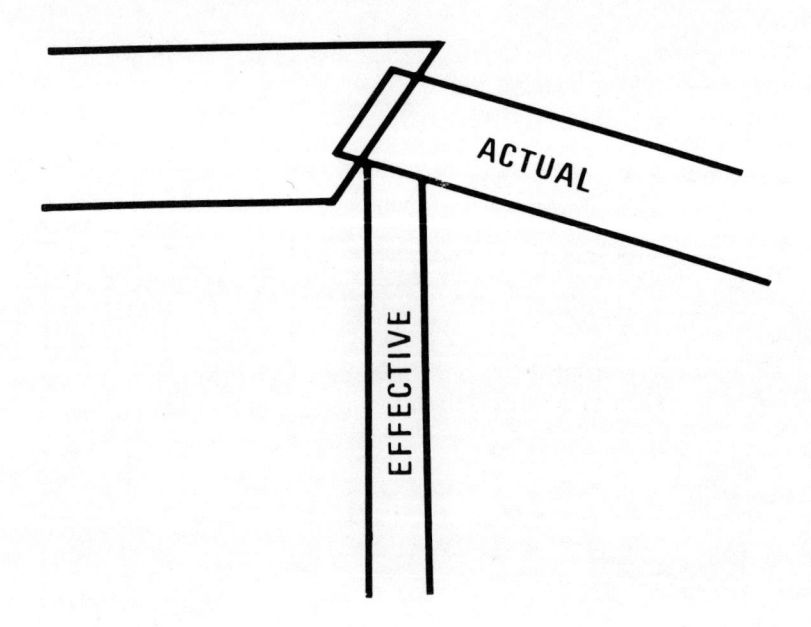

Effective Focal Spot

effective half-life
The half-life of a radioisotope in a biological organism, resulting from a combination of radioactive decay and biological elimination.

effective value
See *root-mean-square value.*

effective voltage
The value of alternating current that will do the same work as its corresponding value of direct current. The effective voltage is 0.707 times the maximum voltage.

electric
Pertaining to electricity or electrical.

electric current
See *current.*

electric field
The electrically sensitive zone around a charged conductor or charged body.

electric field strength
Magnitude of force of an electric field.

electric flux
An electrically sensitive zone that exists around the electrical lines of force.

electric generator
See *generator.*

electrical
Related to or associated with electricity.

electrical capacitor
See *capacitor.*

electrical condenser
See *capacitor.*

electrical contact
See *contact, electrical.*

electrical resistance
See *resistance.*

electricity
A science dealing with the laws and nature of electric charges.

electricity concepts
A.C. and D.C.—A.C. meaning alternating current electrons moving in one direction, then reversing to the opposite direction, as the sine-wave. D.C. meaning direct current, electrons moving in one direction.
Current and static—Current electricity and static electricity referring to electrons in motion is current, and at rest, static.
Positive and negative electricity—Positive referring to proton, the smallest measurable quantity of positive electricity. Negative referring to electron, the smallest measurable quantity of negative electricity.

electric lines of force
Electrical lines that exist around current in motion.

electric motor
See *motor*.

electrification
Process of adding and removing of an electron to and from a body of matter. The methods of electrification are as follows:
Friction—Removing electrons from one object to another by rubbing them together.
Contact—Body charged by friction touches an uncharged object, the latter will also become charged.
Induction—A charged object has a zone around it that has the ability to move electrons in a metallic uncharged object.

electrode
A terminal by which electricity flows from one medium to another.

electrodynamics
Branch of physics that deals with dynamic or moving electric charges.

electrodynamometer
A meter that reads the voltage and amperage of alternating current.

electrolyte
A paste or liquid conducting material in which the flow of electric current takes place by ion migration.

electromagnet
A coil of wire wound around a soft iron core. The core is strongly magnetized when current is flowing and is demagnetized when current stops.

electromagnetic
Pertaining to the combined electric and magnetic fields associated with movement of electrons through conductors.

electromagnetic energy
Energy associated with cosmic, gamma, roentgen, ultraviolet, visible light, infrared, and radio or electric waves.

electromagnetic field
The magnetic field produced around an electromagnet.

electromagnetic induction
Passing a conductor through a magnetic field; its inductive strength depending on the following:
Speed of the conductor.
Strength of the magnetic field.
Angle of the conductor.
Number of windings of the conductor.

electromagnetic spectrum
The total range of wavelengths or frequencies of electromagnetic radiation, extending from the shortest cosmic ray to the longest radio wave. See illustration.

COSMIC	GAMMA	ROENTGEN	ULTRA VIOLET	VISIBLE LIGHT	INFRA RED	RADIO

Electromagnetic Spectrum

electromagnetic unit
An obsolete system of electrical units.

electromagnetic wave
Wave-like shaped lines having an upper and lower peak with a distance between each peak. These waves travel at the speed of light (186,000 miles per second) and are equal to the frequency of vibration (peak of the waves). X-rays are electromagnetic waves and this is called the *Maxwell Theory*.

electromagnetism
The branch of physics that deals with the relationship between electricity and magnetism.

electromotive force (emf)
The electrical pressure that exists in a circuit. Usually called *voltage*, but also called *potential difference.*

electron
Smallest measureable quantity of negative electricity. Negative particle of an atom.

electron beam
The ray of electrons that travel from cathode to anode in an x-ray or valve tube. Also called *cathode rays.*

electron beam tube
Primarily refers to the x-ray tube.

electron cloud
See *thermionic emission.*

electron flow
A current produced by the movement of free electrons toward a positive terminal.

electronic
Pertaining to electron devices or to circuits or systems utilizing electron devices, including electron tubes, transistors, and other devices that do the work of electron tubes.

electronic circuit
Circuit containing one or more electron tubes, transistors, or other devices providing comparable functions.

electronic device
A piece of equipment that uses circuits containing electron tubes, transistors, or other devices that do the work of electron tubes.

electronic subtraction
Method used to provide a subtracted image electronically.

electronic timer
A timer that uses an electronic circuit to operate a relay at a predetermined interval of time after the circuit is energized, as in timing exposure for radiographic equipment range from 1/30 to 20 seconds.

electron linear accelerator
See *linear accelerator*.

electron radiography
The "Xonics" system, a nonsilver method that functions primarily through the ionization of xenon gas with x-rays. A visible image is produced by placing a transparent support in the gas chamber during exposure and later introducing it to either powder cloud development or a liquid toner process.

electron theory
Used since 1950, theories that electrons flow from the overabundance (negative) terminal through the circuit to the deficiency (positive) terminal. Before 1950, the conventional theory was used to describe electricity flow. See illustration.

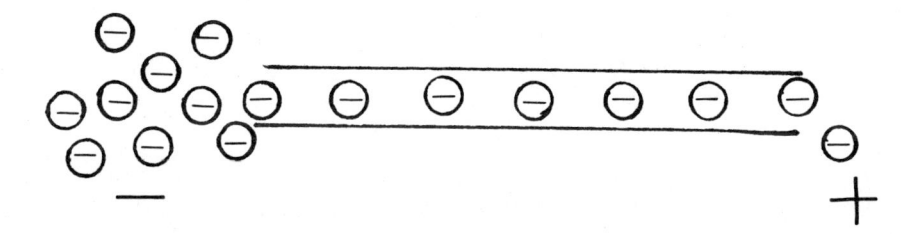

Electron Theory   Electrons flowing from an excess to a deficiency of electrons.

electron tube
An electron device in which conduction of electricity is by electrons moving through a vacuum. For example x-ray, valve, phototiming, and electronic tubes.

electron-volt (ev)
A unit of energy equal to the energy acquired by an electron when it passes through a potential difference of one volt in a vacuum.

electroscope
An instrument for detecting electrical changes. The most commonly used type is a handmade device with a metal rod with two gold leaves at its end in an insulated glass jar. When a charge is enforced upon the rod, the charge passes down the rod and separates the leaf at an angle.

electrostatic induction
Process of charging an object electrically by bringing it near another charged object.

electrostatic laws
There are five electrostatic laws, referring to charges at rest; they are as follows:
- Electrons will gather at the sharpest point of a conductor.
- Like charges repel; unlike attract each other.
- Force between two charges is directly proportional in magnitude and inversely proportional in distance.
- Charges reside only at the external surface.
- Only electrons can move in a solid conductor.

electrostatics
Electricity at rest is static electricity.

electrostatic unit (esu)
Unit used in the electrostatic system that is the charge repelling an exactly similar charge.

element
A category of atoms all of the same atomic number.

Elon
A part of the developing agent referred to as metol. Elon is a trade name of Eastman Kodak. See *metol*.

emission
Any radiation of energy by means of electromagnetic waves.

emulsion, x-ray film
Consists of silver bromide suspended in gelatin. A small amount of sodium iodide may be added. The emulsion is coated on both sides of a polyester plastic base.

energy
The ability to do actual or potential work. The two main types of mechanical energy are:
- Kinetic—energy in motion, and
- Potential—energy at rest.

Energy may be transferred from one form to another, but cannot be created or destroyed.

energy conservation law
See *Law of Conservation of Energy*.

energy dependence
The characteristic response of a radiation detector to a given range of radiation detector to a given range of radiation energies or wave lengths compared with the response of a standard free-air chamber.

envelope
Glass housing of the x-ray or rectifying tube. The glass envelope of the x-ray tube is made from Pyrex because Pyrex can tolerate high temperatures.

equilibrium
The point of balance between two forces.

equivalent roentgen
See *roentgen equivalent physical.*

erg
The absolute centimeter-gram-second unit of energy and work. It is the work done when a force of one dyne is applied through a distance of one centimeter.

erythema
An abnormal redness of the skin due to distension of the capillaries with blood. It can be caused by heat, drugs, ultraviolet rays, or ionizing radiation.

evaporation of filament
Because of prolonged use, the filament diameter becomes thinner and as the diameter decreases, the electrical resistance increases.

excitation
The addition of energy to a system thereby transferring it from its ground state to an excited state. Excitation of a nucleus, an atom, or a molecule can result from absorption of photons or from inelastic collisions with other particles.

excited state
When an electron is missing from an atom, this is called an excited state.

exit dose
The amount of radiation left over after it has passed through the object. Also called *remnant radiation.*

exposure
The quantity of radiation needed for density on a given radiograph, expressed in mA.S. (milliamperage-per-second). The following formula is used:
$$mA. \times Time\ Exposure.\ (S)$$

exposure dose
A measure of x-ray or gamma radiation at a point, based on its ability to produce ionization. The unit of exposure dose is the roentgen.

exposure-dose rate
The exposure dose per unit time. The unit of exposure-dose rate is the roentgen per unit time.

exposure meter
An ionization chamber (Victoreen R-meter) that records directly in milli-roentgens cumulative exposure to x-radiation.

exposure time
The amount of time designated for a given amount of mA. at a set Kv.P. that is used to produce an optimum radiography. Time may be expressed in fractions or decimals and affects density.

exposure timer
An impulse, synchronous, and electronic time device at the control panel to regulate the length of time.

external radiation
The ionizing radiation from a source outside the body.

external circuit
The electrical current supply taken from the armature of a generator.

external surface of conductor
One of the basic laws of electrostatics. Electrons reside at the external areas of a solid conductor because like charges repel each other and there is a greater distance at the outer surface.

Fahrenheit (F)
Thermometric scale on which the freezing point of water is 32° and the boiling point, 212°. Formula for conversion of Fahrenheit to *centigrade*:
$$C = \frac{5}{9}(5 - 32)$$

farad (f)
A unit of electrical capacitance.

fatty meal
Given to patients 30 to 40 minutes prior to gall bladder film for the purpose of contracting the gall bladder.

feet per second (fps)
A unit of speed at which sound waves travel through a medium.

ferromagnetic
Materials having a strong magnetic attraction, for example, iron, cobalt, and nickel.

field
One of the equal parts into which a frame is divided in interlaced scanning

television for x-ray equipment. A field includes one complete scanning separation from top to bottom of the picture and back again. Also see *television field.*

field coil
A coil used to produce a constant-strength magnetic field in an electric motor and generator.

field intensity
See *field strength.*

field of force
A region in space in which force is exerted on electric charges by other stationary or moving charges.

field of view
That area over which a lens can create a usable image. It is frequently measured as an angle.

field size
The area of the body to be irradiated.

field strength
The strength of an electric, magnetic, or electromagnetic field at a point. Also called *field intensity.*

filament
Symbol F. It is at the cathode terminal of the x-ray or valve tube and is enclosed along with the anode in a glass tube. The filament of a tube, when heated to incandescence, emits electrons. The rate of emission of electrons, is controlled by a low-voltage heating current, in a process termed thermionic emission and is controlled by the predetermined milliamperage. See illustration.

filament circuit
The circuit that supplies the current to the filament of the x-ray tube for heating purposes. It consists of the variable resistor, filament ammeter, step-down transformer, and filament of the x-ray tube. The circuit operates at approximately 3/5 amperes and 5/15 volts.

filament current
A term for the temperature of the filament of the x-ray tube and measured in amperes.

filament emission
Liberation of electrons from a heated filament wire in an x-ray or valve tube. See *thermionic emission.*

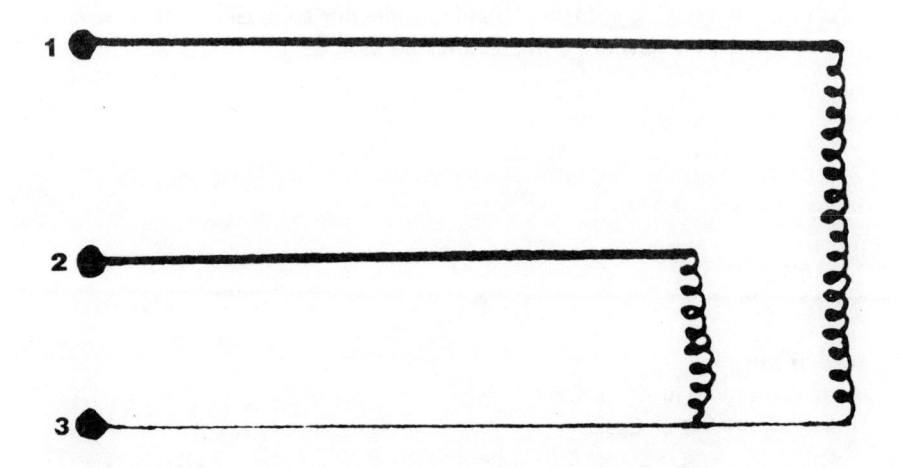

Filament Wire #1 supplies low voltage to the large filament; #2 supplies low voltage to the small filament; and # 3 is the high-voltage wire common to wires #1 and #2.

filament saturation
See *saturation current*.

filament stabilizer
See *stabilizer, filament*.

filament transformer
A step-down transformer used exclusively to supply current for the filament of x-ray, valve, and electron tubes. For the x-ray circuit, the filament transformer works simultaneously with the choke coil to vary the tube current (mA.).

filament voltage
The voltage applied to the terminals of the filament in an x-ray, approximately five to 15 volts.

film (x-ray)
A sheet of polyester plastic with emulsion of silver bromides suspended in gelatin, that is mainly sensitive to radiation and light. There are two types of film—nonscreen and screen. Nonscreen film is sensitive to direct radiation and screen film is sensitive to blue light emitted from intensifying screens, but this type can be used with direct radiation.

film badge
A badge containing a piece of unexposed x-ray film, worn on the person as a means of measuring radiation exposure. The badge has different metal so it may record radiation variation. The films are removed from time to time, developed, and the resulting emulsion density measured to determine exposure.

film base
See *base, x-ray film.*

film bin
A drawer container subdivided by vertical partitions for the use of storing different sizes of opened x-ray film boxes. The drawer is counterweighted so that when it is opened, it will stay open, and with a light touch, it will close automatically. This container must not be opened when lights are on.

film contrast
See *characteristic curve.*

film corner cutter
A mechanical device that trims rough corners, made by the clips from the film hanger.

film emulsion
See *emulsion, x-ray film.*

film graininess
See *graininess, film.*

film hangers
Frame-like holders constructed of stainless steel to accommodate various sizes of films. The x-ray film is clipped to each corner of this frame, then placed into the developer, fixer, wash, and dryer. It is removed from the hanger and the rough corners are trimmed with a corner cutter.

film ring
A film badge in the form of a finger ring.

film sensitivity
See *speed, film.*

film speed
See *speed, film.*

film-screen contact test tool
A 14 x 17 inch frame-like device with wire mesh housed in plastic that is placed on top of a cassette to demonstrate film-screen contact.

filter, radiography
A piece of metal (such as aluminum) placed in the path of a diagnostic x-ray beam to reduce soft rays and skin exposure. The aluminum is generally 2 mm. thick.

filter, safelight
See *safelight lamp*.

filter, therapy
The exposure rate is reduced and the quality is enhanced by adding filters to the therapy beam. The half value layer (HVL) is that material (usually a metal) that reduces the beam by half the original value, the metal referring to a filter.

filtration
Removal of some components of a heterogenous beam of x-ray and other radiation by inserting various metals into the beam path.

fixation, x-ray film
A process that removes the unexposed and undeveloped silver halides, and preserves and hardens the film image.

fixer (hypo) solution, x-ray
The purpose of the solution is to remove the unexposed and undeveloped silver halides, and preserve and harden the film's image. The fixing agent is sodium thiosulfate (powder) or ammonium thiosulfate (liquid); preservative is sodium sulfite; hardener is chrome alum or potassium alum; and neutralizer is sulfuric acid or acetic acid.

flat film
A somewhat controversial term applied to certain x-ray examinations of the abdomen, with different connotations in various radiology offices. There is no universal agreement whether the term is limited to prone, supine, or upright projection, nor is there agreement whether AP or PA projections are the routine.

flat plate
Referring to glass plates used in the early years of x-ray. This term is now obsolete because the glass plates have not been used since the 1920s. We now record radiographic images on the film developed by George Eastman. Other terms that are sometimes used are plain film, scout film, and preliminary film.

floppy disk
A flexible vinyl disk, approximately 8 inches in diameter, on which digital information can be recorded magnetically. It can be used for archival storage for the electronic CT image.

fluorescence
The emission of light from crystals of certain substances, such as barium platinacyanide, calcium tungstate, and rare earth, which will glow when struck by x-rays.

fluorescent screen
A sheet of material coated with a fluorescent substance that emits visible light when irradiated with ionizing radiation.

fluorography
A form of radiography of an image produced on a fluorescent screen and recording a radiographic image.

fluorometer
An instrument that measures the intensity of x-rays and other radiation by measuring the intensity of the fluorescence produced.

flurometry
Measurement of the intensity of radiation.

fluoroscope
A piece of x-ray equipment usually having an x-ray tube beneath the x-ray table and a fluorescent screen above the table parallel to the tube. The patient is placed between the tube and the screen; the operator controls the radiation from behind the screen. A fluorescent screen used with an x-ray images is interposed between the x-ray tube and the screen.

fluoroscopic
Pertaining to *fluoroscopy*.

fluoroscopic examination
A radiographic procedure using the fluoroscope to examine and permanently record the radiographic image on film emulsion.

fluoroscopic image
A variety of densities shown on the fluoroscopic screen as the radiation passes through the patient.

fluoroscopic image intensifier
See *image intensifier*.

fluoroscopic timer
A hand-setting timer, usually set at five minutes, that will shut off the current after the time has elapsed.

fluoroscopy
The use of a fluoroscope for an x-ray examination.

fluoroscopy chair
An obsolete lead back chair that faces the fluoroscopy screen; the operator straddles the seat to face the patient.

flux
See *electric flux*.

"F" number
See *relative aperture*.

focal-film distance (F.F.D.)
The distance from the focal spot of the x-ray tube to the x-ray film. Same as *T.F.D.—target-film distance*.

focal length
A property of all lenses. That distance from the lens at which the lens will image an infinitely distant object.

focal plane
Area of interest. In tomography, that part of the body that appears in focus.

focal spot (target)
The small area on the target of the anode of an x-ray tube that gives off x-rays when hit by the electron stream. The smaller the focal spot, the greater the geometric definition.

focus object distance (F.O.D.)
The distance from the focal spot of the x-ray tube to the object being radiographed.

focusing cup
Along with the filament, the focusing cup determines the size and shape of the target (focal) spot. The cup is constructed of molybdenum.

focused grid
A grid with angulated lead strips so that the strips converge or are focused upon a definite point at the same distance from the grid, this point being the x-ray tube focusing spot. See illustration.

focusing radiographic
Centering the central ray (x-ray beam) to the field of interest.

fog
See *light, x-ray exposure, chemical,* and *age*.

force
Refers to the push or pull of work.
Force × Distance = Work.

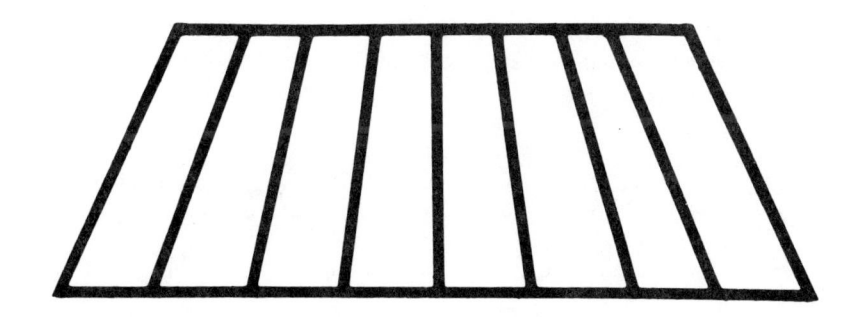

Focused Grid

four-valve-tube rectification
See *full-wave rectification*.

frame
See *television frame*.

frame rate
In cine or television cameras, that number per unit of time (usually one second) during which sequential pictures are displayed.

free air ionization chamber
See *Victoreen R-meter*.

free electron
Electrons at the outermost shells of atoms. Little or no energy is needed to liberate them.

frequency
Symbol f. The number of complete cycles per unit of time for a periodic quantity such as alternating current, sound waves, or x-rays. Frequency is usually expressed in cycles.

friction marks
Artifacts on the x-ray film due to discharge of static electricity.

frilling
Defect in a radiograph associated with separation of the emulsion from the base at the margin of the film.

fulcrum
In tomography, the pivot point or axis of rotation for the x-ray tube and the film tray.

full-wave rectification
Electrically changing alternating current so that the impulses go in only one direction during both half-cycles by means of valve or rectifying tubes. Also called *bridge circuit* and *four-valve-tube rectification*. See illustration.

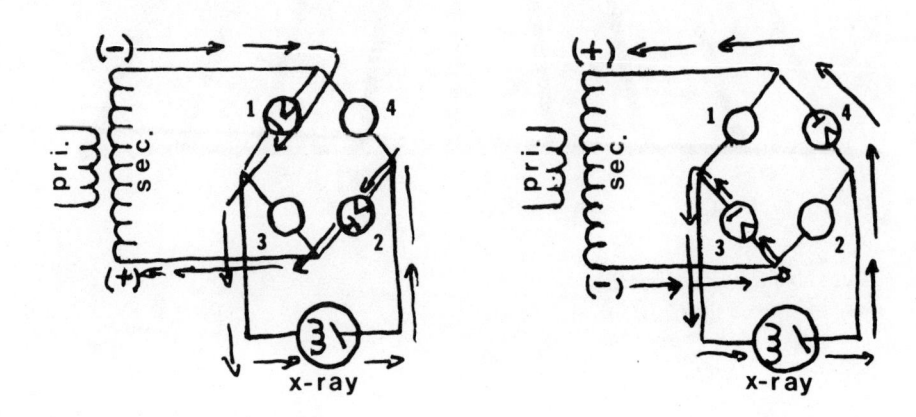

Full-wave Rectification The commonly used wiring system operating with four valve tubes. Valve tubes #1 and #2 rectify positive alternation, whereas #3 and #4 rectify the inverse alternation.

fuse
Symbol *F*. A protective device containing a short length of special wire that melts when the current going through it exceeds the rated value for a given period of time. A fuse is inserted in series with the circuit being protected, for example, at the main switch of the x-ray circuit.

fusion, nuclear
Combination of two or more atomic nuclei.

gadolinium and lanthanum
Phosphors that absorb more of the available x-ray photons and have a higher conversion efficiency to light than does calcium tungstate, the phosphor most commonly used in intensifying screens. Sometimes referred to as *rare earth*.

gain curve, ultrasound
The gain curve is set to allow the proper amplification of the echoes that have been attenuated by body tissue. Sometimes referred to as the *amplification system*.

gallon
A unit of liquid measurement equal to four quarts. Processing tank capacity is

referred to in gallons, using the formula:

$$\frac{\text{width} \times \text{length} \times \text{depth less one inch}}{231 \text{ (cubic inches per gallon)}}$$

galvanometer
An instrument for indicating or measuring a small electric current by means of a mechanical motion derived from electromagnetic or electrodynamic forces produced by the current.

gamma, film
This is the slope of the straight line portion of the characteristic (H&D) curve.

gamma camera
A device that records the gamma radiation emitted by a scanning agent localized in that organ.

gamma cascade
Successive gamma transitions occurring in radioactive transformations.

gamma emitter
An atom whose radioactive decay process involves the emission of gamma rays.

gamma heating
Heating resulting from absorption of gamma-ray energy by a material.

gamma radiation
Radiation of *gamma rays*.

gamma radiography
Radiography by means of *gamma rays*.

gamma-ray counter
A radiation counter designed for detecting and recording the intensity of gamma rays.

gamma-ray level indicator
A level indicator in which the rising level of the liquid or other material reduces the amount of radiation passing from a gamma-ray source through the container to a Geiger counter or other radiation detector.

gamma rays
Electromagnetic radiation emitted from radioactive materials. They are characteristically similar to roentgen rays but more penetrating than alpha or beta.

gamma-ray spectrometer
An instrument that measures the energy distribution of gamma rays.

gammas
See *gamma rays*.

gamma scanning
The scanning of a fuel rod in a nuclear reactor for gamma activity by moving the rod past a slit in a lead block. Photons emerging from the slit are detected by a sodium iodide scintillation spectrometer and recorded as a function of rod position.

gantry
The movable frame on a CT machine that holds the x-ray tube, collimators, and the detectors.

gap
A break in a closed magnetic circuit, containing only air or filled with a non-magnetic material. The spacing between two electric contacts. See *air gap*.

gassy tube
A vacuum tube (x-ray or valve tube) that has not been fully evacuated or has lost part of its vacuum due to damage. Also called *soft tube*. If an x-ray tube is gassy, the mA. or mA.S. meter will fluctuate during the exposure.

GBX filter
Kodak safelight filter which can be used with all blue- and most green-sensitive film. Illumination comparable to *Wratten 6B*.

Geiger counter
A radiation counter instrument that uses a Geiger counter tube to count ionizing particles, such as cosmic-ray particles. Each particle ionizes the gas in the tube in such a way that the total ionization per event is independent of the energy of the ionizing particle. Also called *Geiger-Mueller counter*.

Geiger-Mueller counter (G-M counter)
See *Geiger counter*.

gelatin
A suspending material consisting of silver bromides made from cattle skin and mustard oil for sensitivity of film emulsion.

general effect of radiation
Exposure to radiation that has harmful effect on blood-forming organs, such as bone marrow and lymphatic tissues.

general radiation
Referring to "white" radiation or brems radiation. General radiation constitutes

90 percent of the emitted x-rays in the diagnostic range; the remaining 10 percent of the emitted x-rays are characteristic radiation.

generating equipment, x-ray
See *x-ray generator.*

generator
Symbol *G*. Electrical device that converts mechanical energy into electrical energy. Also called *dynamo.*

generator rule
See *left-hand rule.*

genetic effect of radiation
Exposure to radiation that has harmful effects on future generations. This results from the vulnerability of the genes, particularly chromosomes of sex cells, to radiation damage.

geometric detail
The radiograph's sharp image, even though that image may be over- or under-exposed, over- or under-penetrated.

geometry, plane
Branch of mathematics that deals with figures in one plane. There are five divisions: straight line, rectangle, square, triangle, and circle.

glove (lead protection)
Protective gloves for radiology, have approximately .5mm. lead equivalent.

glutaraldehyde
A hardener added to the developer of the automatic processing chemicals.

G-M counter
See *Geiger counter.*

graininess
A mottling of the radiographic image.

graininess, film
The clumping of the emulsion of a radiographic film. The slower the film speed the finer the grain and the less visible emulsion clumping on the finished radiograph. The graininess is too small to give serious consideration. However, because of the various speeds of radiographic film, it does contribute to radiographic mottle.

-gram
Data of which is written or recorded.

gram-rad
A unit of integral absorbed dose of radiation, equal to 100 ergs per gram.

graph
A drawing showing the relationship between two quantities, one depending on the other.

-graphy
Referring to that which writes or describes.

gray scale (of an image)
Refers to the number of gray tones (which are distinguishable to the eye) in going from the blackest black to the whitest white.

grenz rays
Radiation of long-wave length of one to 10 angstroms, produced by using a special x-ray tube operating at five to 15 Kv.P. (kilovoltage peak). Named by Dr. Gustave Bucky in 1929.

grid, electronic
Symbol G. An electrode located between the cathode and anode of an x-ray tube and serving to control the flow of electrons from cathode to anode.

grid focus
The point at which all of the radiopaque strips in a grid would meet if they were extended.

grid lines
Linear lines recorded on a finished radiograph from the Bucky diaphragm because the bucky did not move during exposure or failed to follow the recommended grid radius. See illustration.

grid, radiographic
A radiographic device constructed of radiolucent material between lead strips for the prime purpose of cleaning up scatter and secondary radiation. It is placed between the patient and the x-ray film. See *parallel grid*, *focused grid*, and *stationary grid*. See illustration.

grid radius
The distance between the x-ray tube focus and the grid.

Grid Lines

DISTANCE BETWEEN LEAD STRIPS

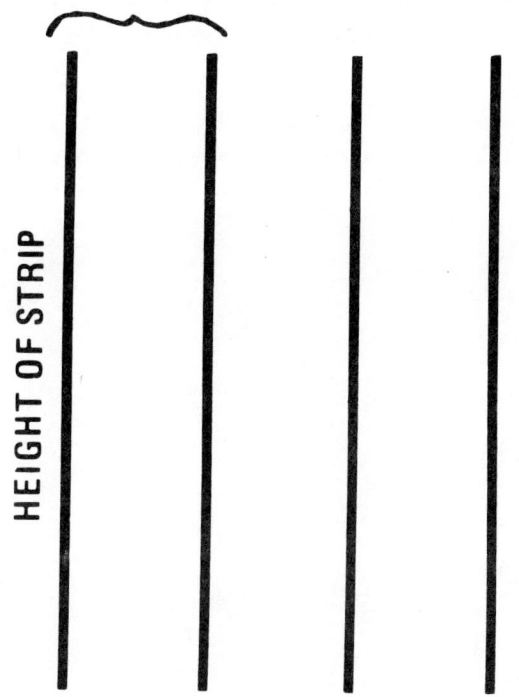

HEIGHT OF STRIP

Grid, Radiographic

grid ratio
The relationship between the height of the lead strips and the width of the radiolucent (nonopaque) material between them.

ground
A conductor wire connected to the highest voltage point of the x-ray equipment and to the ground or earth to prevent any electrical shock. Any overabundance of electrons can then flow to ground and any deficiency of electrons can then be taken from ground.

ground state
The state of a nucleus, atom, or molecule at its lowest energy. All other states are "excited."

ground wire
A conductor used to connect electric equipment to a ground rod or other grounded object.

grows up
Term that refers to the *emf* of the magnetic field expanding around the conductor.

guide shoe marks
Evenly spaced lines (or marks) occurring during the film transport, appearing as either plus or minus density in nature. They are caused by the guide shoe adjustment on the automatic processor's developer rack having been set too close to the adjacent roller.

Gyratome
The Xonics tomographic and radiographic system offering linear, circular, and trispiral tomography along with routine radiographic capabilities.

halation
The unsharpness of an image that may accrue when duplicating a film. The light source that passes through the original radiograph may reflect back onto the copy.

half-cycle
The time interval corresponding to half a cycle or 180° at the operating frequency of a circuit or device.

half-life (HL)
The average time required for one-half the given time of radioactive materials disintegration to expire. Also called *half-value period*.

half-value layer
The thickness of a material (usually metal) when introduced in the path of radiation, will reduce the intensity of radiation to half of the initial value. Also called *half-value thickness*.

half-wave rectification
Rectification in which current flows only during the positive impulse or alternation of a sine wave. See illustration.

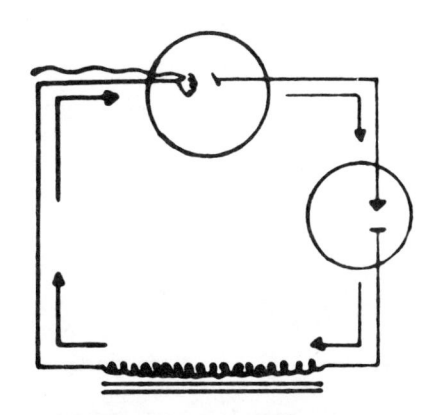

Half-wave rectification with one valve tube.

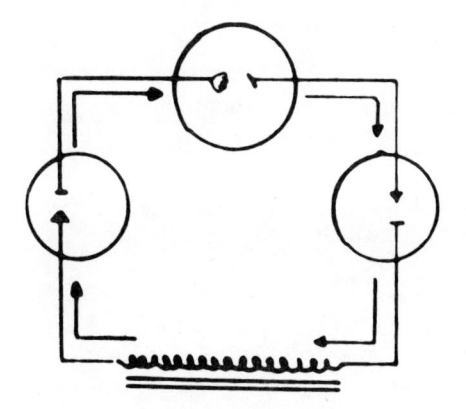

Half-wave rectification with two valve tube.

Half-wave Rectification

halides
Compounds of metals with halogen elements: bromine, chlorine, and iodine.

handbooks of protection
The National Bureau of Standards, Washington, D.C., prepared four inexpensive handbooks for those individuals working with x-rays or radiation. They are:

33—Medical X-ray and Gamma Ray Protection for Energies up to 10MeV
51—Radiological Monitoring: Methods and Instruments
59—Permissible Dose from External Sources of Ionizing Radiation
73—Protection Against Radiations From Sealed Gamma Sources
76—X-ray Protection Up to Three Million Volts.

H and D curve
A characteristic curve of a photographic emulsion obtained by plotting film density against the logarithm of the exposure. Also called Hurter and Driffield curve—named after the British scientists founders.

hangers
See *film hangers*.

hard copy, CT
Any permanent or semi-permanent medium containing information that will remain relatively unchanged until some specific action or erasure is used. Typewritten printouts, photographs, magnetic tape, and magnetic disk recordings are considered hard copy. See *archival storage*.

hardness, radiographic
The penetrating ability of x-rays. The shorter the wavelength, the harder the radiation and the greater its penetrating ability.

hard steel
Used in the manufacturing of permanent magnets because of its characteristics of low permeability and high retentivity.

hard x-ray (radiation)
An x-ray having high penetrating power, this being achieved by high Kv.P., and radiographically resulting in a long scale contrast.

harmful effect, radiation
Any amount of radiation, no matter how small, has a harmful effect on living tissues.

head clamp
A mechanical device attached to the x-ray unit in which the patient's head is held during a radiographic examination in order to reduce motion.

heat
See *thermal radiation.*

heat dissipation
The ability of the x-ray tube anode to conduct heat away from the target by air, oil, or water colling system.

heat exchanger
A device used to circulate and cool the oil of the x-ray tube housing for the purpose of increasing the heat-storing capacity and cooling rate of the housing.

heat unit (H.U.)
Measurement of the quantity of heat deposited in the anode of an x-ray tube. Determined by the formula:

Kv.P. × mA. × time (single phase); Kv.P. × mA. × time × 1.35 (three phase, six pulse); and Kv.P. × mA. × time × 1.41 (three phase, twelve pulse).

heel effect
The heel effect refers to the unequal intensity of the x-ray beam, the intensity being greatest on the cathode side of the beam and least intense on the anode side of the beam. Some of this variation is reduced by use of lead apertures and shutters that limit the periphery of the primary x-ray beam. See illustration.

helix
A bedspring-shaped coil of wire. One of the basic parts of an electromagnet. See *electromagnet.*

hertz (Hz)
European term for *cycles per second.*

hesitation marks
These marks occur in automatic processors when the developer transport rack is malfunctioning or when someone temporarily shuts off the processor's transport system while film is in the developer solution. The hesitation marks will appear as a plus or minus density line running in a 90° angle to the direction of film traveling in an irregular pattern.

heterogeneous, x-rays
Radiation having unlike wavelengths. This radiation occurs when using a single-phase generator.

high tension (voltage)
Thousands of volts that are commonly called high voltage transformers.

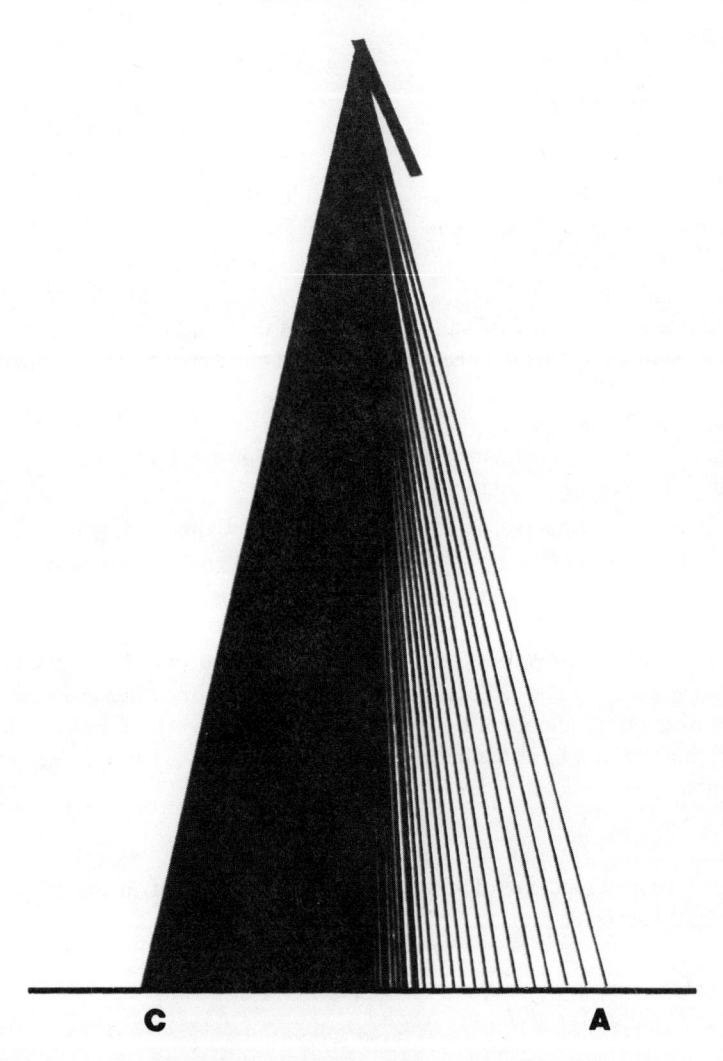

Heel Effect   There is more density on the cathode side "C" of the reflected target of the x-ray tube.

high vacuum
A degree of vacuum at which essentially no gases or vapors are present.

high voltage transformer
A step-up transformer, having less conductor turns on the primary (low voltage) side and more conductor turns on the secondary (high voltage) side. Also called the *x-ray transformer.*

homogeneous radiation
Radiation having a narrow band of frequencies and like wavelengths. This radiation occurs when using three-phase generating x-ray equipment.

hot
An informal word meaning *radioactive*.

hot cathode x-ray tube
A cathode from which electrons are emitted by heating the filament. Invented by W.D. Coolidge, General Electric Company Laboratories, in 1913. Also called *thermionic cathode*.

hot spot
A term used for therapy technologists when referring to overlying treatment areas by two portal openings. See illustration.

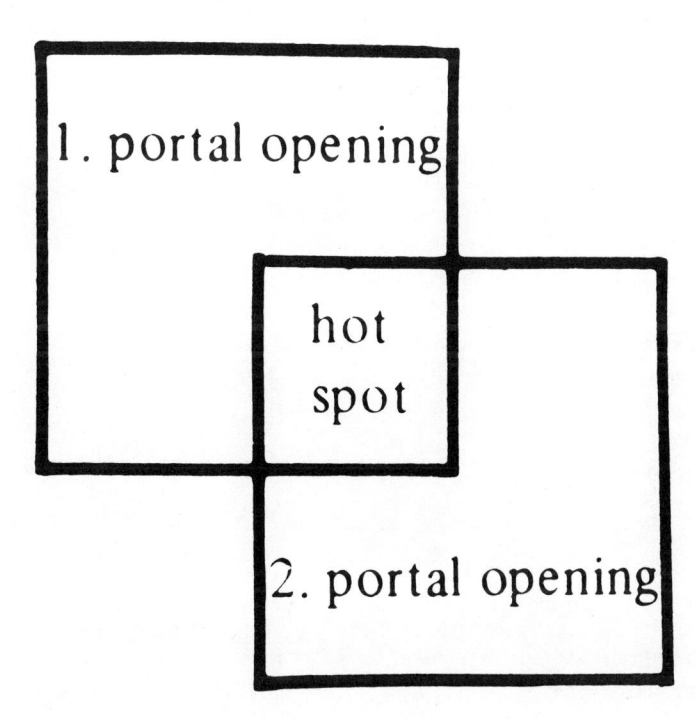

Hot Spot

hot wire
A conductor carrying current.

Hounsfield units (H)
A specific range of CT numbers based on using water as the zero reference value, with air placed at -1000 units and dense bone at +1000 units.

hydrogen
Symbol *H*. The simplest of all the 103 elements having one known atom, consisting of only one proton and one electron.

hydrometer
A sealed glass tube designed to float in a solution and used to determine overconcentration or dilution of mixed chemistry.

hydroquinone
A part of the developing agent that acts slower during the development and produces the density and contrast to a desired level of a radiograph. Metol is also a part of the developer agent and works in the early stages of development.

hypo
See *fixer solution*.

hyposulphite of soda
May be added to fixer to clear and fix the film emulsion. Not listed as one of the major chemicals for fixer solution.

hysteresis loss
A minimal power loss in an iron-core transformer. A.C. builds up magnetic domain first in one direction, then in another. This rearrangement causes heat in the iron core. It can be reduced by using silicon steel.

$I^2 \times R$ = watts
Power consumed formula.

illuminator
A device used for film viewing. This may be a single or multipanel device.

image
An optical counterpart of an object as a real image on photographic or radiographic film emulsion.

image amplifier
See *image intensifier*.

image intensifier
An electronic system of producing flourescent images by amplification of the brightness level so that they may be observed by means of a mirror-optical system or on a television monitor. Viewing may be done in subdued room light and dark adaptation is unnecessary.

image intensifier tube
An evacuated electronic tube capable of converting an imput beam of x-ray energy into a visible light image of increased brightness. Typical tubes have input screen diameters of six or nine inches.

impedance
Symbol Z. The opposition offered by a component or circuit to the flow of an alternating or varying current. Impedance is expressed in ohms. The formula is not beneficial for radiological purposes.

implant, therapeutic radiology
To insert radioactive material in a needle or other container, into the effective area, as a form of treatment.

impulse
Meaning pulse or alternation. See *alternation*.

impulse timer
Operates at 1/120 to 1/5 second, this being precise timing system. This type of timer counts impulses of the alternating currents at the zero point of the sine wave.

incandescence
Heating of the filament to "boil off" electrons. See *thermionic emission*.

inductance
Symbol L. The property of a circuit that opposes a charge current flow of an inductance circuit. Referred to as bucking or inductive reactance. Measured in henrys.

inductance—capacitance (LC)
Containing both inductance and capacitance, as provided by coils and capacitors.

induction
The process of inferring the same charge on an uncharged object by bringing it into the magnetic field zone.

induction coil
The purpose is to increase voltages. It is constructed of a primary conductor coil, having fewer turns, and a secondary conductor coil, having many more turns. Both the primary and the secondary coil are wound around an iron core and highly insulated from each other. May be referred to as a *transformer*.

induction motor
An a.c. motor in which a primary winding, the stator, is connected to the power source, and a secondary winding, the rotor, carries induced current. This type of motor is used for rotating the anode of rotating anode x-ray tubes. See illustration.

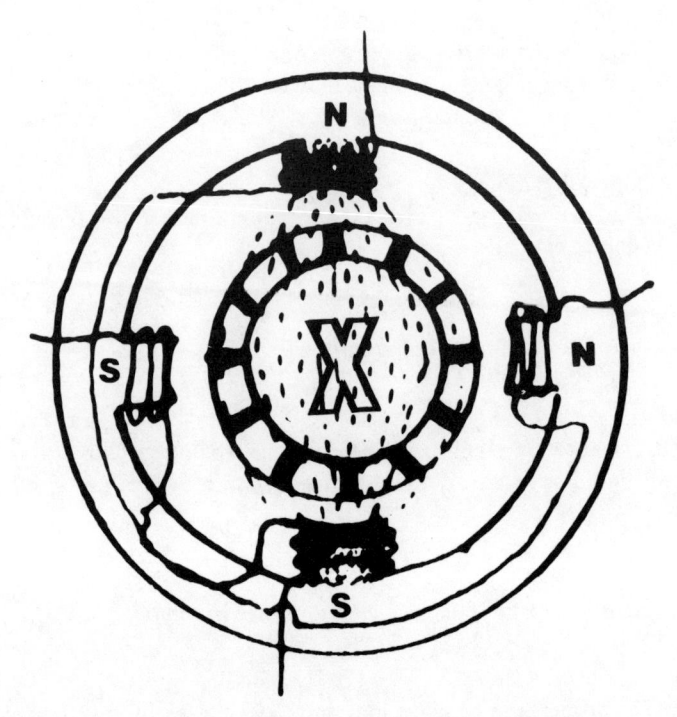

Induction Motor Two magnetic flux fields that rotate the rotor "X."

inductive
Pertaining to *inductance*.

inductive reactance
Symbol X_L. Because of the persistently changing magnetic field around the coil of wire using a.c., there is a back emf in one direction, then in another; this is inductive reactance or bucking.

inductor generator
An a.c. generator in which all the windings are fixed and the flux linkages are varied by rotating an appropriately toothed ferromagnetic rotor.

industrial radiography
Radiography of castings, welded joints, and other industrial products for quality control and flaw detection.

inertia
A property of matter whereby a body at rest will stay at rest and a body in motion will stay in motion until acted upon by some outside force.

infrared radiation
Radiation in the electromagnetic spectrum shorter than radio wave but longer than visible light, ranging in wave length from .1 cm to 8000Å.

inherent
Built into the object, part of the essential material.

inherent filtration
Filtration introduced by the wall of an x-ray tube and permanent tube housing enclosure. Equivalent to .5mm aluminum.

inherent resistance
Resistance that is present in copper conductors or various electrical devices.

in-phase
Two or more items or components, usually having some periodic mode of operation, operating exactly in synchronism.

input
The terminal to which the power is applied.

input side
The primary coil of a transformer or electrical device.

installation
The act of placing a complete x-ray equipped unit. Each unit or x-ray room is referred to as an installation.

instantaneous radiation
The radiation emitted during the fission process. Frequently called prompt gamma rays or prompt neutrons. Most of the fission products continue to emit radiation after the fission process.

insulated
Separated from other conducting surfaces by a nonconducting material.

insulation
A material having high electric resistance suitable for separating adjacent conductors in an electric circuit.

insulator
A device having high electrical resistance, used to prevent undesired flow of current from the conductors to other objects. Material such as rubber, oil, glass, dry wood, and bakelite, have an atomic valance full with electrons, permitting no electron movement.

integral dose
A calculated dose for a portion of the body, determined by the size of the field, the skin dose, and the depth of tissue at which the dose falls to one-half the skin dose. Generally measured in roentgens (R). Also called integral absorbed dose and volume dose.

integral timer
A timer connected in the circuit of an x-ray machine that adds up the exposu to determine a total amount of time.

intensify
To increase the brilliance of the object's image projected on the output phosphor of an intensifier tube.

Intensifying (Intensification) Factor
The ratio of the exposure required without intensifying screens to the exposur required without intensifying screens to the exposure required with intensifyir screens to achieve equal blackening of radiographic films. Another name for th term is *speed factor* and is expressed by:

$$IF = \frac{\text{exposure without screens}}{\text{exposure with screens}}$$

intensifying screens
Paired screens composed of fluorescent crystals, that are sandwiched close to the radiographic film and inhoused into a radiographic cassette.

intensity, electrical
Symbol I. The strength of current of an electrical circuit. Intensity is sometim interchangable with current or amperage.

intensity, radiation
Refers to the concentration or quantity of x-rays striking an area per unit of time.

interface
Boundary zone or wall between two different media or tissues, for example, the wall of the urinary bladder against the wall of the uterus.

interlace
Term used when referring to television radiography for the production of lines on the television screen.

interlock
Several types of interlocks may be found in a radiology department, each

serving to prevent the operation of a unit until a necessary safety precaution has been observed.

internal conversion
A form of radioactive decay.

internal radiation hazard
Those individuals who have been exposed to radioactive materials deposited within their body, for example, radium watch dial painters.

internal resistance
See *inherent resistance.*

Inverse square law of radiation
The intensity or exposure rate of radiation at a given distance from the source is inversely proportional to the square of the distance. See illustration.

Formula: $\dfrac{I_1}{I_2} = \dfrac{d_2}{d_1}^{2}$

inverse voltage
The negative impulse or alternation of the sine wave.

involuntary motion
The uncontrolled physiological function of the human body organs.

ion
A charged atom. A negative ion has gained one or more extra electrons, whereas a positive ion has lost one or more electrons.

ion chamber
See *ionization chamber.*

ion pair
A positive ion and an equal-charge negative ion, usually an electron, that are produced by the action of radiation on a neutral atom or molecule.

ionic polar valence
See *chemical bond.*

ionic solution
A chemical solution made up of sodium and chlorine, which are brought together to produce a direct current source, such as a battery.

ionization
The process by which an atom gains or loses an electron, thereby acquiring a

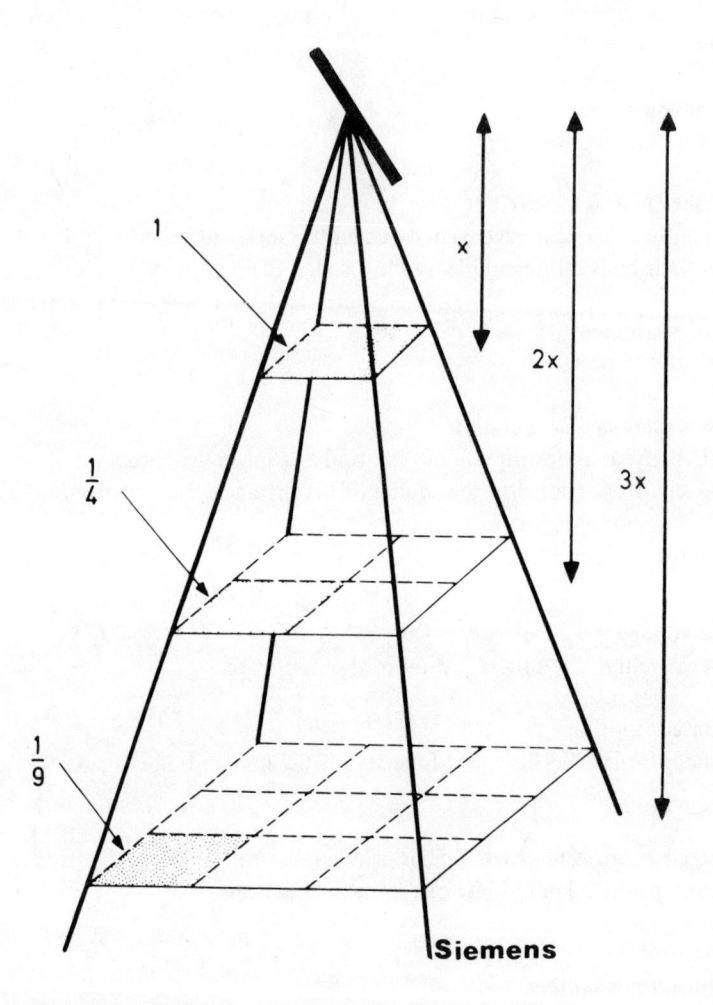

Inverse Square Law of Radiation When the distance is doubled, there is one-fourth the amount of radiation, and when the distance is tripled, there is one-ninth the amount of radiation.

total charge and becoming an ion. Ionization may be produced by radiation and by many other means.

ionization chamber
A chamber containing two oppositely charged electrodes in a gas. When the chamber is exposed to radiation, the gas is ionized and each ion is drawn to the electrode of opposite polarity. The resulting current through the chamber is proportional to the intensity of the exposed radiation.

ionization instrument
An ionization chamber used to measure the intensity of ionizing radiation.

ionization potential
That quantity of energy, expressed in electron volts, required to remove an electron from a neutral atom.

ionizing radiation
Radiation or radioactive particles that have sufficient energy to produce ionization directly in their passage through air.

iron
See *soft iron*.

iron core
See *core iron*.

iron-core transformer
A transformer in which the iron-core makes up part of the path for the magnetic lines of force to be concentrated for the emf.

irradiated
Describing areas that have been exposed to any form of radiation.

irradiation
The exposure of a material, object, or patient to ionizing radiation.

isobar
An atom with the same atomic weight but different atomic number.

isocentric mounting
An arrangement making it possible to move a radiation source easily about a treatment site while maintaining a fixed distance and beam angulation.

isodose chart
A chart showing distribution of depth dose produced by irradiation.

isotope
Atoms having the same number of nuclear protons (equal to the atomic number) but different numbers of nuclear neutrons.

isotopic mass
Obsolete term for *atomic mass*.

isotopic number
See *neutron excess*.

isotopy (isotopism)
The phenomenon that deals with isotopes.

joint, electrical
A juncture of two wires or conductive paths for current. Permanent joints are soldered, whereas temporary joints are held together by spring slips or screws.

joule
A unit of energy or work. One joule is equal to 1 watt-second. Named in honor of James B. Joule.

juice
Slang term for *current*.

jumper
A short length of conductor used to make a connection between two points of a circuit.

K electron
An electron having an orbit in the K shell, which is the first shell of electrons surrounding the atom's nucleus.

Kenotron tube
The General Electric Company's term for valve or rectifier tube.

Kilo-(KO)
A prefix representing 1000.

Kilocurie (Kc)
One thousand curies.

Kilocycle (Kc)
One thousand cycles. Interpreted as meaning thousands of cycles per second.

Kilo-electron-volt (Kev)
One thousand electron-volts. It is the energy acquired by an electron that has been accelerated through a voltage difference of 1000 volts.

Kilohm (K or Kohm)
One thousand ohms. Thus, 15K is 15,000 ohms.

Kilometer (Km)
One thousand meters, or 3,280 feet.

Kilosecond
One thousand seconds.

Kilovolt (Kv)
One thousand volts of electrical pressure.

Kilovolt-Ampere (Kv.A.)
Rating form for alternating current generators (instead of kilowatts); determined by the formula:

$$Kv. \times I = Kv.A.$$

Kilovoltage
A voltage of the order of thousands of volts, such as the voltage applied to an x-ray tube. Penetrating power of x-ray beam.

kilovoltmeter
A voltmeter the scale of which is calibrated to indicate voltage in kilovolts. See *prereading kilovoltmeter.*

kilovolt peak (Kv.P.)
The peak (maximum) voltage applied to an x-ray tube.

Kilowatt (Kw)
One thousand watts.

kinescope
The display or picture tube of the monitor.

kinetic energy
Energy associated with motion.

Kirchhoff's Law
The algebraic sum of the currents that meet at any point of a circuit is zero.

K line
One of the characteristic lines of an atom. It is produced by excitation of the electrons in the K shell.

K radiation
The x-ray radiation emitted when K electrons are excited.

K shell
The innermost layer of electrons surrounding the atom's nucleus, having electrons characterized by the principal quantum number 1.

kymograph
A device for radiographically recording the range of motion of various organs, especially the chambers of the heart throughout the cardiac cycle. The method by which this is done is called kymography.

kymoscope
An x-ray apparatus used in viewing kymographic films.

labyrinth
A doorless passageway constructed so that a complete U turn must be traveled before entering a doorless opening to the darkroom. See illustration.

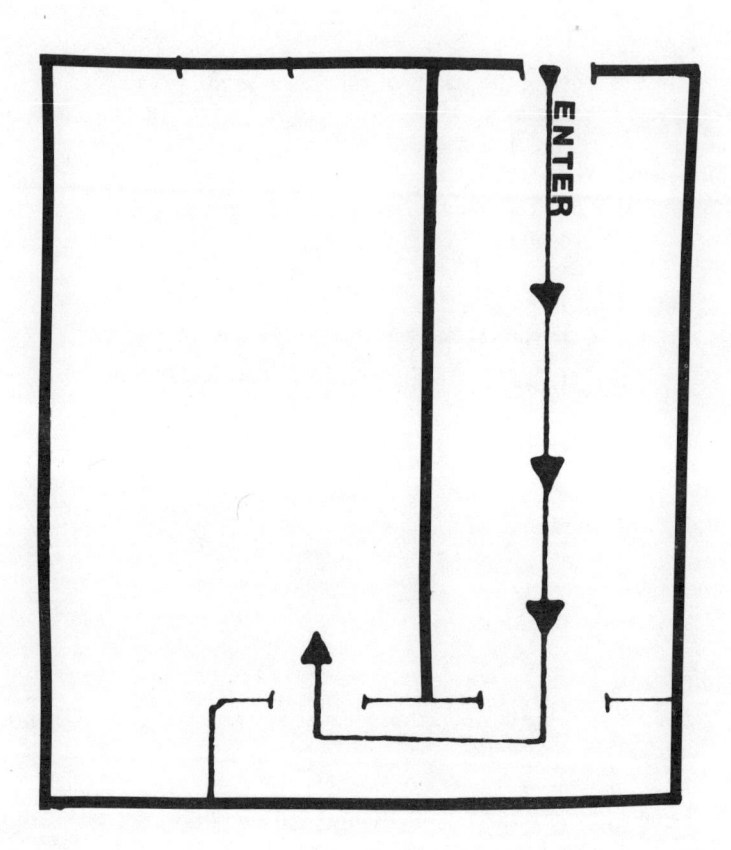

Labyrinth

lag
See *screen lag*.

laminagraphy
See *body section radiography*.

laminated core
The core material of transformers are laminated (layered) to minimize eddy current. See *eddy current*.

laminated silicon steel plates
Lamination of the iron core of a transformer using silicon steel plates insulated from each other with varnish to minimize eddy current.

lanthanum oxybromide and terbium
Fluorescent materials used in the manufacture of intensifying screens.

latent image
A stored or invisible image produced by film emulsion by x-ray or light energy, that becomes a visible image upon development.

latent period
The interval between irradiation and the appearance of the image upon development.

latitude, density
The milliampere-second has density latitude that is not strongly critical when incorrect mA.S. is used. This is due to the fact that most x-ray film has latitude. That range of density (mA.S.) within a given radiographic exposure that is not strongly influenced.

latitude, radiographic
The range in exposure factors that will produce a diagnostic radiographic image; the extent of variation between maximum and minimum density in a radiograph consistent with the diagnostic quality of the radiograph; free from limits, long scale latitude means less contrast.

latitude, x-ray film
The ability of film emulsion to record radiographic images with a long range of gray tones.

Law of Conservation of Energy
Energy cannot be created or destroyed, but can be changed from one form to another.

law of electric charges
Like charges repel; unlike charges attract.

law of inverse square
See *inverse square law*.

laws of magnetism
The three fundamental laws of magnetism are:
- Every magnet has a north and south pole.
- Like poles repel; unlike poles attract.
- The force of attraction or repulsion between two magnetic poles is directly proportional in strength, and inversely proportional to the square of distance between them.

lead
Symbol *Pb*. A soft gray metallic element used as a shielding material in x-ray work. Atomic number is 82.

lead apron
See *apron*.

lead equivalent
The amount of lead required to reduce radiation as the material in question.

lead glass
Lead impregnated glass window of the control booth, employed to protect the operator from radiation.

lead gloves
See *gloves*.

lead protective chair
See *fluoroscopy chair*.

lead rubber
Lead impregnated rubber that can be used for apron and gloves because of its pliability.

leak, electrical
In an electric capacitor or condenser that stores electrical energy on the insulated surface of the parallel plates, an escape or leak of energy may occur. This loss or leak of energy cannot be corrected and the replacement of the capacitor is necessary.

leakage radiation
Radiation from anything other than the intended radiating system. A common example is electromagnetic radiation that escapes through defects in shielding.

leaky, capacitor
Capacitor in which the resistance has dropped below its normal value so that excessive leakage current flows.

left-hand rule
For a movable current-carrying wire or an electron beam in a magnetic field: If the thumb, first, and second fingers of the left hand are extended at right angles to one another, with the first finger representing the direction of magnetic lines of force and the second finger representing the direction of electrons, the thumb will be pointing in the direction of motion of the wire. Also called *rule* or *dynamo rule*. See illustration.

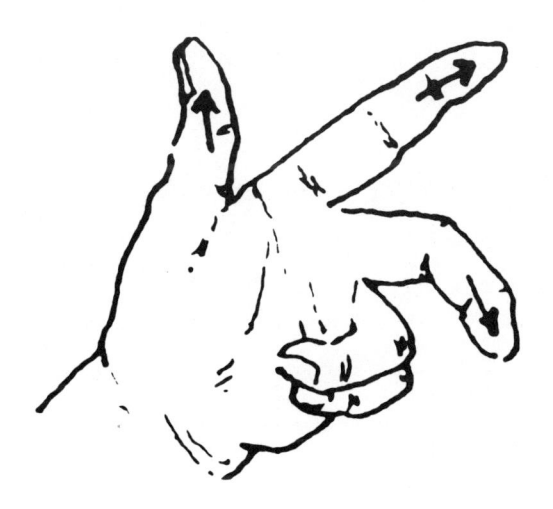

Left-hand Rule

left-hand thumb rule
If the wire is grasped in the left hand so that the thumb points in the direction of the electron flow (- to +), the fingers encircling the wire will indicate the direction of the magnetic lines of force around the wire. See illustration.

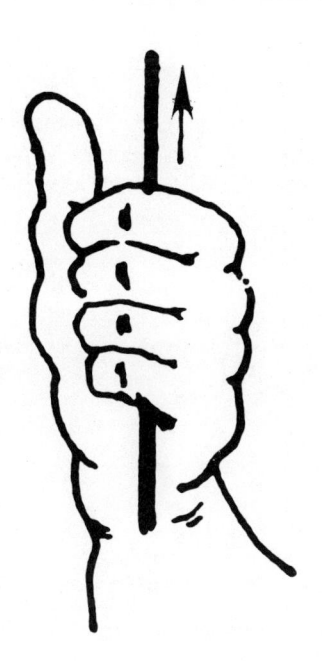

Left-hand Thumb Rule

L electron
An electron having an orbit in the L shell, which is the second shell of electrons surrounding the atom's nucleus.

Lenard ray tube
A cathode ray tube used in 1892 (before x-ray discovery) by Philipp Lenard.

lens
In television and photographic cameras, a highly corrected set of optical elements in a mount. Used to form an image of the subject on some light-sensitive surface for reproduction.

lens axis
The line defined by connecting the curvature centers of all the lens elements.

lens speed
See *relative aperture*.

lethal dose (LD)
A dose of ionizing radiation sufficient to cause death.

lifetime
See *half-life*.

light
Electromagnetic radiation having wavelengths capable of causing the sensation of vision, ranging approximately from 4,000 angstroms to 7,700 angstroms. The velocity of light is 186,000 miles per second. Also called *light wave*.

light fog
Fog density that appears on a finished radiograph. This may occur when the darkroom is not lightproof; film holders are cracked; light bulb power is too large; safelight filter is cracked; safelight series is incorrect; film is exposed too long to safelight filter; distance to safelight is too short; there are many other minor causes, as well.

light trap
See *labyrinth*.

linear
Like a line or straight.

linear accelerator
A machine arranged to move electrons in a straight line up to energies in the range of three to 24 Mev; used in medical and industrial research.

linear attenuation coefficient
The ratio of change of x-ray beam intensity through a uniform material of unit length (parallel to the x-ray beam) in comparison to a prescribed attenuation standard.

linear electron accelerator
See *linear accelerator.*

linear energy transfer (L.E.T.)
The linear rate of energy loss (locally absorbed) by an ionizing particle traversing a material medium, expressed usually in Kev.

linear grid
Same as *parallel.*

linear scanning, ultrasound
Scanning system in which the transducer moves the form of the body in a straight line and the direction of the beam is not changed.

line drop
See *voltage drop, line voltage compensator,* and *automatic line voltage compensator.*

line-focus principle
Referring to the anode of a diagnostic tube. If you were lying supine and looking upward at the target, the focal spot (effective) would be a smaller spot, rather than the actual rectangle, which it is. In other words, the actual focal spot is 2mm. × 4mm. and the effective focal spot is 2mm. × 2mm.

line pair
A means of expressing resolution or resolving power.

line voltage
The main voltage of the electric current that enters the radiology department. See *line voltage compensator* and *automatic line voltage compensator.*

line voltage compensator
A switch that is connected to the incoming electrical line of the x-ray circuit and is placed in parallel across the greater part of the autotransformer. See *manually controlled line voltage compensator* and *automatic line voltage compensator.*

liter
A measure of volume of the metric system.

L line
One of the characteristic lines of an atom. It is produced by excitation of the electron in the L shell.

load, electrical
The amount of electric power that is drawn from a power line, generator, or other power source.

load (loading) capacity
Referring to the heat tolerance of an x-ray tube.

local effect of radiation
Exposure to radiation that has harmful effects to skin (erythema) and may produce cataract formation on the eye lens.

lodestone
A natural magnetic ore consisting of iron and oxide.

logarithms
It is the power or number that will raise the base ten to a given quantity. Logarithms are used in sensitometry to compress large quantities of data into a small numerical graph.

long (low) scale contrast
Effected by higher Kv.P. range, produces nine to 14 varieties of blacks and whites. The resulting radiograph has complete penetration with all areas visible.

loss
Power that is dissipated in a device or system without useful work. See *transformer loss.*

low voltage current
Refers to the filament current for the x-ray tube circuit.

low-voltage therapy x-rays
Voltage ranging from 50 to 120 Kv.P. More frequently called superficial therapy. This type of treatment is used mainly for lesions of the skin.

L shell
The second layer of electrons surrounding the nucleus of an atom, having electrons whose principal quantum number is 2.

luminescence
Emission of radiation or light from a substance as a result of previous action

of some form of energy, for example, the glow of light from phosphorus after exposure to sunlight.

Lysholm grid
A stationary grid of fine lead strips used with the Potter-Bucky diaphragm, invented by Erik Lysholm, a Swedish radiologist.

magnet
A material that has magnetic properties, such as iron. A permanent magnet will produce a permanent magnetic field, whereas an electromagnet possesses magnetic properties only when current is flowing through its windings.

magnetic domain
The polarity of attraction inside a magnetic bar that lines up from north to south. See illustration.

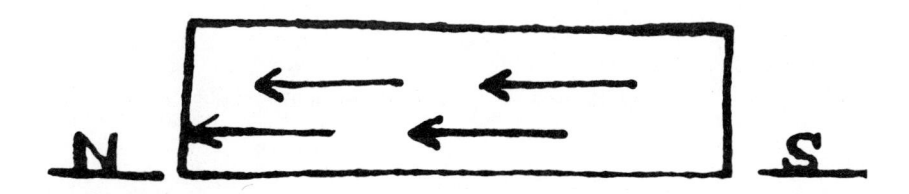

Magnetic Domain

magnetic field
The region in which a magnetic force exists around a charged magnet.

magnetic field strength
The magnitude of the magnetic field around a charged magnet.

magnetic flux
Magnetic sensitive zone that exists around the magnetic lines of force.

magnetic force
See *magnetic field strength*.

magnetic induction
When a nonmagnetized iron is brought near a magnet, the iron will become magnetized. This process is called magnetic induction.

magnetic lines of force
Magnetic strength that exists around a charged magnet.

magnetic material
A material that shows magnetic properties. Ferromagnetic materials are strongly magnetic—for example, iron, cobalt, and nickel.

magnetic permeability
Ease with which a given material can become magnetic.

magnetic pole
One of the two poles of a magnet near which the magnetic intensity is greatest. These poles are known as north and south.

magnetic recording
A means of obtaining a permanent record of an electrical signal. Converts the signal to a magnetic field that is used to magnetize permanently some storage medium. Common devices are video tape recorders and video disk recorders.

magnetic retentivity
The ability of a given material to hold a magnetic charge.

magnetics
The branch of science that deals with magnetic (magnetism) phenomena.

magnetism
A property possessed by iron, steel, and other magnetic materials, wherein these materials can produce magnetic lines of force capable of interacting with electrical fields or magnetic fields.

magnification factor (MF)
This is the ratio of the body width to the object width recorded on x-ray film. The formula is:

$$\text{magnification factor} = \frac{\text{image width}}{\text{object width}}$$

or:
$$MF = \frac{TDF}{OFD}$$

magnification percentage
This is the percentage of enlargement of the image as compared with the object, and is not a true ratio. The formula is:

$$\text{percentage magnification} = \frac{\text{image width} - \text{object width}}{\text{object width}}$$

magnification, radiographic
The enlargement or distortion of a radiographic image recorded on film emul-

sion, can be minimized by reducing the object-film distance, and increasing the focus-film distance.

magnitude of ripple
The distance between one peak to the following peak of the sine wave of any rectified current. See *ripple, electrical.*

main gain control, ultrasound
Refers to the input/output control, dampening control, and so on. This controls the ability to penetrate the patient.

main switch
This is usually a double-blade, single-throw switch; when the switch is closed, the alternating current flows to the x-ray machine.

"make"
Referring to the instant the switch is closed or current switch is turned on. "Making contact."

mammography film
A single-emulsion film characterized by high contrast, slow speed, and fine grain. There are several types of mammography film available for low dose systems.

Mammomat
The Siemens mammographic unit which may use nonscreen film, film/screen combinations, or xeroradiography.

Mammorex
The Picker mammographic system designed to meet the needs of breast imaging.

manifest image
That visible image upon development of a radiograph.

manually controlled line voltage compensator
A device to adjust the incoming line voltage manually by adjusting a meter found at the control panel. It is placed in parallel with the autotransformer. See illustration.

mask(s)
Lead shield(s) used to limit the arena of exposure to the film and reduce scatter.

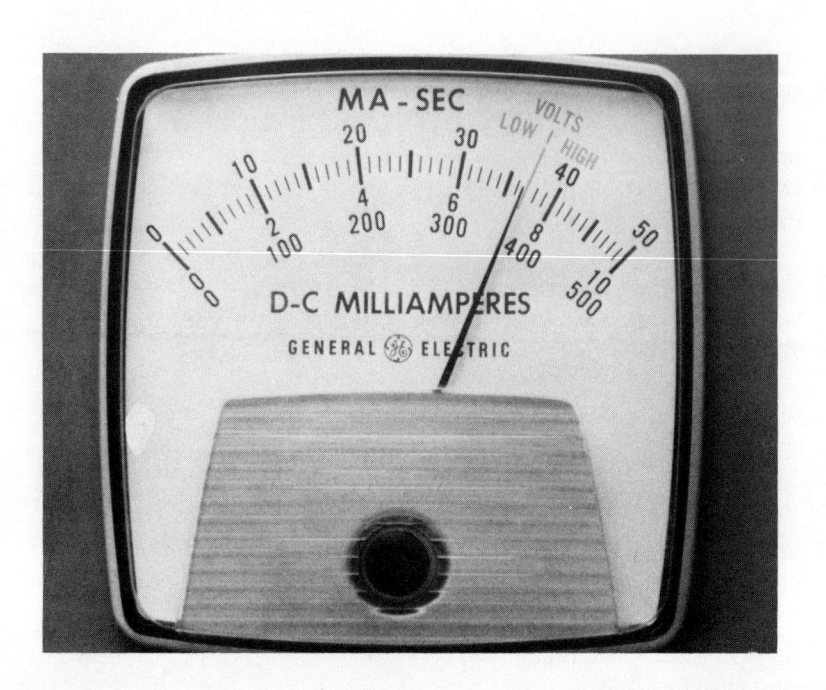

Manually Controlled Line Voltage Compensator

mass
The weight of matter of a body.

mass number
The number of protons and neutrons in the nucleus. Same as atomic weight or atomic mass.

matrix
A system used to divide an area into equal segments of uniform size, with all segments spaced equidistantly. The matrix pattern is defined by the number of vertical columns versus the same number of horizontal rows.

matter
Anything that occupies space and has weight. Matter may be gaseous, liquid, or solid, and usually is electrically neutral.

maximum current
The value of alternating current that will do the same work as the corresponding value of direct current. The maximum current is 1.41 times the effective current.

maximum permissible dose (MPD)
For radiation workers 5R per year is permissible. The MPD formula is:

MPD = 5(N-18) = Rads or Rems

Five represents the permitted yearly dose. N represents the individual's present age. Eighteen represents the 18 years of the individual's life when he was not exposed to radiation.

maximum voltage
The value of alternating current that will do the same work as the corresponding value of direct current. The maximum voltage is 1.41 times the effective voltage.

Maxwell Theory of Radiation
Radiation is electromagnetic waves with wavelengths and frequencies of vibrations, traveling with the speed of light, and having no electrical charge. Contradictory is the photon or quantum theory. See *photon theory of radiation.*

maze
An interlocking two-door system to provide a safe and convenient entrance into the darkroom. As one door opens, the other door remains locked until the first door closes and vice versa.

mean deviation, CT
The average, or arithmetic-mean of the deviation, taken without regard to sign, from some fixed value. The mean deviation is expressed as a CT number(s) with respect to a specified material, the CT number of which is used as the standard (or fixed) value.

mean life
See *half-life.*

mechanical energy
See *x-ray generator.*

mega (abbreviated M)
A prefix representing 10^6, or one million.

mega-electron-volts (Mev)
Million electron-volts.

M electron
An electron having an orbit in the M shell, the third shell of electrons surrounding the atomic nucleus, counting out from the nucleus.

metallic silver
The density on a finished radiograph is referred to as metallic silver.

meter-kilogram-second
Metric system meaning meter-length, kilogram-mass, and second-time.

metol
A part of the developing agent; acts during the early stages of development; produces the basic gray image of a radiograph. Hydroquinone, which is also a part of the developer agent, works slower than metol.

micro
A prefix representing 10^{-6} or one-millionth.

microcurie
One-millionth of a curie.

microfarad
One-millionth of a farad.

microfilm
A miniature film for record keeping for the convenience of space saving, at times recorded on 35 mm photographic film.

micromicro
A prefix representing one-millionth of a millionth. Now called *pico* or 10^{-12}.

micron
Symbol M. A unit of length. The thousandth part of one millimeter.

microradiography
The radiography of small objects having details too fine to be seen by the unaided eye, with optical enlargement of the resulting negative.

milli-(m)
A prefix representing 10^{-3}, or one ten-thousandth.

milliammeter
An ammeter whose scale is calibrated to indicate current values in milliamperes.

milliampere (mA)
One-thousandth of an ampere.

milliampere-seconds (mA.S.)
The product of time (sec) of an x-ray exposure and the milliamperage (mA) used. The mA.S. determines the quantity of radiation that is produced by an exposure.

millicurie (mc)
One-thousandth of a curie.

millimeter (mm)
One-thousandth of a meter.

million electron volt (Mev)
Former name for *mega-electron-volt*.

millirad (mrad)
One-thousandth of a rad.

millirem (mrem)
One-thousandth of a rem.

milliroentgen (mr)
One-thousandth of a roentgen.

millisecond (msec)
One-thousandth of a second.

minification
This word is used in reference to the smallness of the image on the output screen (one inch diameter) from the input screen (nine inch diameter).

minimum exposure, radiography, and fluoroscopy
To minimize radiation exposure for the obvious reasons, the following recommendations should be observed: maximum collimation; filtration by 3mm al.; high speed intensifying screens; lead shielding of gonads; recommended kilovoltage; well-trained radiographer.

mixture
Single kind of matter having a varied composition.

M line
One of the characteristic lines of an atom. It is produced by excitation of the electrons of the M shell.

mobile intensifier
An integrated system of x-ray generator, x-ray tube, and image intensifier. A self-contained unit that may be moved readily to different locations.

mobility
The degree of motion of an organ or structure.

modulate
To regulate or modify some process by means of an external influence or signal. In a television system, it has to do with varying the intensity in the kinescope—accomplished by modulating its electron beam with the signal from the television camera.

molecule
Smallest subdivision of a substance having the physical properties of that substance. It can be either simple (like an atom) or compound (unlike an atom).

molybdenum
Symbol *Mo*. A metallic element, used for the focusing cup of the x-ray tube. Atomic number is 42.

monitor
A television screen that displays the radiographic image.

mono-
Prefix meaning one.

monochromatic radiation
Electromagnetic radiation having a single wavelength, or photons all having the same energy.

monocular stereoscope
A hand-held portable stereoscopic unit, extremely small and lightweight.

monoenergetic radiation
Radiation consisting of particles having the same energy.

motion image
Voluntary motion is the unwillingness or inability of the patient to follow the technologists instructions to hold still.
Involuntary motion is the uncontrolled physiological functioning of the human body organs.

motor, electrical
A device that converts electrical energy to mechanical energy.

mottle, radiographic
The product of screen mottle and film graininess.

mottle, screen
It is caused by the built-in structure of the screen phosphor coating. Screen mottle appears as an unevenness or spotty effect. See *mottle, radiographic*.

moving bucky
A reciprocating or synchronizing grid which moves during the exposure time.

M shell
The third layer of electrons about the nucleus of an atom, having electrons characterized by the principal quantum number 3.

multiformat camera
A means of recording CT, Ultrasound, and Nuclear Medicine procedures usually on "8×10" film using various formats.

multiphase
An electrical current having many phases, for example, three-phase generator.

multiphase generator
See *three-phase generator*.

multisection cassette
Used for tomographic studies permitting a visual radiographic record of several films placed in one cassette and taken with one exposure.

mutual inductance
Symbol *M*. A measure of the amount of inductive that exists between two coils.

mutual induction
When current is flowing through one (primary) coil and the second (secondary) coil is placed near the first (primary) coil, current will flow through the second coil if it is crossed by the changing (a.c.) magnetic lines of force; this is known as mutual induction.

mylographic stop
A myelographic stop is a mechanical device used in conjunction with myelographic examinations in order that the fluoroscopy equipment not touch or displace the needle in place for the lumbar puncture.

Mylar
Trademark of DuPont for their x-ray film base.

NaI (Sodium Iodide)
A scintillator crystal that converts x-rays into light. It is used as a detector in many CT machines.

natural magnet
See *lodestone*.

neck, x-ray tube
The small tubular part of the envelope of an x-ray tube, extending from the funnel to the base and housing.

negative
A terminal or electrode having more electrons than normal. Electrons flow out of the negative terminal of a voltage source.

negative charge
Condition of the atom in which it has more electrons than normal.

negative direction
Negative alternation, impulse, or pulse of the sine wave.

negative electron
An electron, as distinguished from a positive electron or positron. Also called *negatron*.

negative ion
Atom having an excess electron.

negative terminal
The negative (-) terminal of a battery that has more electrons than normal. Electrons flow from the negative terminal through the external circuit to the positive terminal.

negatron
Product of pair production and is nothing more than a free electron. It can join the atom.

N electron
An electron having an orbit in the N shell, which is the fourth shell of electrons surrounding the atomic nucleus, counting out from the nucleus.

net density
That density above base density or fog (0.25) and is produced by the exposure.

neutral atom
An atom in which the number of positive charges in the nucleus is equal to the number of electrons that surround the nucleus.

neutron
Smallest quantity of neutral electricity found in the nucleus of an atom.

neutron excess
The number of neutrons in a nucleus in excess of the number of protons.

neutron number
Symbol N. The number of neutrons in the nucleus of an atom.

no connection
Symbol NC. Two wires that cross each other but are not connected.

noise
An undesired electric disturbance that blurs out useful visible information on the television monitor of image intensification.

nonconductor
See *dielectric*.

nonlinear
Not directly proportional, not straight.

nonmagnetic
Not magnetizable, and hence, not affected by magnetic fields. Examples are air, glass, paper, and wood.

nonradio-opague
Easily penetrated—for example, wood.

nonscreen film
Also called direct-exposure film. Film that depends mainly on direct x-ray exposure, and should be used for nonscreen radiographic exposures. This film is about four times as fast as screen film, therefore, requires one-fourth the exposure of screen film for equal radiographic density.

nonscreen holder
An x-ray film holder having no screens and that is used for nonscreen radiographic work. See illustration.

nonvisualization
Failure to visualize an organ on radiographic film or record radiographic sharpness of an image.

normal temperature and pressure
Standard condition—$0°C$. and 76 cm water pressure.

north pole
The pole of a magnet at which magnetic lines of force leave.

N shell
The fourth layer of electrons about the nucleus of an atom, having electrons characterized by the principal quantum number 4.

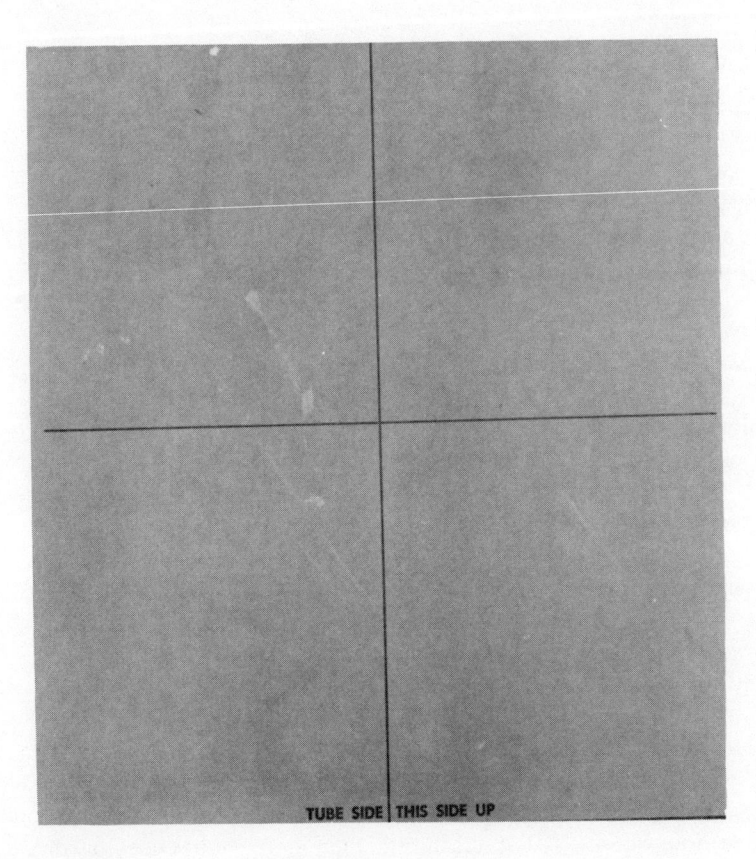

Nonscreen Holder

nuclear emulsion
A photographic emulsion specially designed to register individual tracks of ionizing particles, such as, scan recording.

nuclear energy
Energy released by nuclear fission or nuclear fusion. Also called *atomic energy, atomic power,* or *nuclear power.*

nuclear medicine
The branch of medicine concerned with diagnostic and therapeutic use of radionuclei.

nuclear particle
A particle in the atomic nucleus. It may be either a proton or a neutron. Also called *nucleon.* A particle emitted by an atomic nucleus, such as an alpha particle or a beta particle.

nuclear radiation
The radiation of neutrons, gamma particles, and other particles from an atomic nucleus as a result of nuclear fission or nuclear fusion.

nuclear structure
The internal structure of the atomic nucleus.

nucleus
The central part of an atom, possessing a positive charge and containing nearly all the mass of the atom. The nucleus consists of protons and neutrons, together known as nucleons, except for the hydrogen nucleus, which consists of only one proton. Also called *atomic nucleus.*

nuclide
An atom species of a single atomic number and a single mass number.

object-film distance (OFD)
Distance between the object or skin and the cassette or film.

objective lens
In an image intensifier, the lens that collects the light from the output screen and projects it into the camera lens.

objective plane
See *focal plane.*

octet rule
This rule applies to the semiconductor of the solid-state rectifier, in which the atoms of the semiconductor share their valence of eight electrons. (Octet meaning eight.)

O electron
An electron having an orbit in the O shell, which is the fifth shell of electrons surrounding the atomic nucleus, counting out from the nucleus.

ohm
The unit of electric resistance. It is the resistance through which a current (electrons) of one ampere will flow when a voltage (pressure) of one volt is applied.

ohmmeter
An instrument for measuring electrical resistance. Its scale may be graduated in ohms or megohms.

Ohm's law
The current I in a circuit is directly proportional to the total voltage E in the

circuit and inversely proportional to the total resistance R of the circuit. The law may be expressed in three forms:

$$R = \frac{E}{I} \ ; \ I = \frac{E}{R} \ ; \ E = IXR$$

Where: E = Volt or electromotive force.
         I = Ampere or intensity of electrons
         R = Resistance or slows up electrons and divides voltages. See illustration.

Ohm's Law formula
E=Volt or electromotive force.
I =Ampere or intensity of electrons.
R=Resistance or slows up electrons and divides voltages. See illustration.

Ohm's Law formula

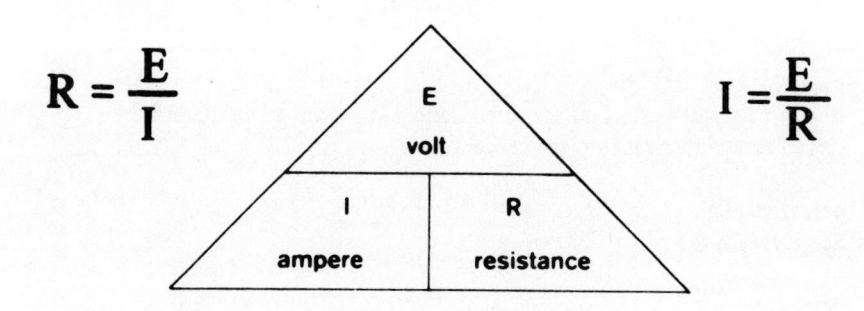

$$R = \frac{E}{I} \qquad\qquad \begin{array}{c} E \\ \text{volt} \\ \hline I \quad|\quad R \\ \text{ampere} \quad \text{resistance} \end{array} \qquad\qquad I = \frac{E}{R}$$

$$E = I \times R$$

Ohm's Law Formula

oil-cooled tube
An electron tube in which the heat produced is dissipated, by means of oil.

opacity
A quality or state of a body that makes it impervious to light.

opaque
Not transparent or translucent.

opaque media
Any contrast media that can be injected or introduced into the body.

open, electrical
A break in a path for electric current.

open circuit
An electric circuit that has been broken so there is no complete path for current flow.

open core transformer
The primary and secondary coils, each highly insulated from the other, are wrapped around a primary and a secondary unconnected iron core.

optics
The branch of science that deals with the phenomena of light and vision.

optimum Kv.P.
A technique of exposure using a fixed Kv.P., as opposed to variable Kv.P.

Optiplanimat
The Siemens automated unit which may be used for planigraphy, zonography, and Bucky radiography in all tilt positions between +110 and -90.

orbit
See *atomic orbit.*

orbital electron
An electron that is moving in an orbit around the nucleus of an atom.

Orbitome
The Picker multidirectional tomographic system designed to do hypocycloidal, trispiral, circular, rectilinear, transverse, longitudinal, and diagonal tomographic slices.

Orbix
The Siemens x-ray unit for survey and precision detail radiography of the skull and small bones of the skeleton in the recumbent or seated position.

Orthicon
A highly sensitive television camera used for fluoroscopic image intensification. One type of television pick-up tube, usually three or four inches in diameter and 15 to 18 inches long. Includes a photo-multiplier section for extreme sensitivity to low levels of light.

ortho
Film that is sensitive to both blue and green light.

orthovoltage therapy radiation
Voltage ranging from 200 to 250 Kv.P. This type of treatment is used mainly for lesions well below the surface of the skin.

oscillating grid
A grid that moves during the exposure. Same as *reciprocating grid.*

oscilloscope
An instrument that traces the design of wavelengths and frequencies.

O shell
The fifth layer of electrons about the nucleus of an atom, having electrons characterized by the principal quantum number 5.

outlet
A power-line termination from which electric power can be obtained by inserting the plug of a line cord. Also called a *receptacle.*

out-of-phase
The opposite of in-phase. The periodic motions do not occur in each component at the same time. One hundred eighty degrees out-of-phase means that at any given time they are exactly opposite. See illustration.

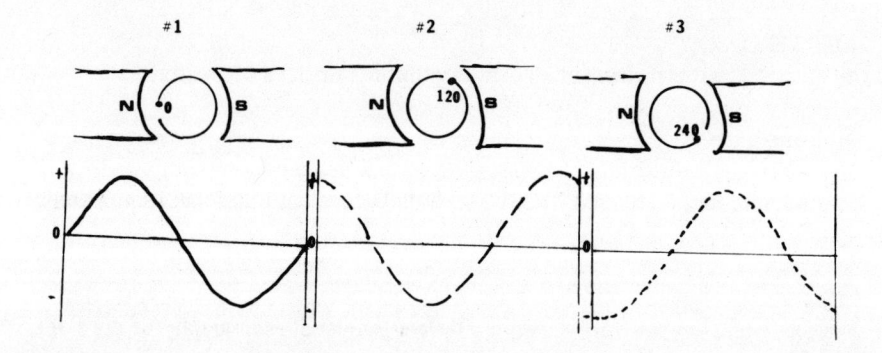

Out-of-phase

output
The useful energy delivered by a circuit or device. The value in R/min. of radiation from an x-ray tube.

output side
The secondary side of a transformer or electrical device.

overdevelopment
Permitting the film to remain in the developer beyond the normal or pre-

set time. This decreases radiographic contrast and increases radiographic density.

overexposure
An excess of time exposure or milliamperage. This decreases radiographic contrast and increases radiographic density.

overhead film
Film taken with the x-ray tube over the x-ray table.

overloading
Exceeding the heat capacity of an x-ray tube. See *heat unit.*

overpenetrated film
A radiograph having an excess of kilovoltage.

oxidation
The process of changing a compound by removing one or more electrons from an atom, ion, or molecule. Oxidation signifies the loss of an electron.

pair production
A megavoltage photon with energy above 1.02 million electron volts that, upon approaching a nucleus, may disappear and give birth to a pair—a negative electron or negatron and a positive electron or positron.

panoramix
Originally designed for dental radiography; this mobile unit produces an umbrella shaped x-ray beam. The tube extends 4½ inches, and can be positioned in any natural body cavity, producing an inside-out radiograph of distortion and elongation, freeing superimposition.

parallax
The apparent displacement or the difference in apparent direction of an object as seen from two different points not on a straight line with the object. See illustration.

parallel circuit
Electrical circuit the component parts of which are in a branch from the main power supply. Its characteristics are: amperage divides or varies; voltage stays the same; and total resistance is always less than the smallest resistor in the circuit. See illustration.

parallel grid
A grid with lead strips placed perpendicularly in assembly so that the projected lead strips will not converge at any point at any distance. This type of grid permits a long target-grid distance but is critical for grid cut-off at distances below 36 inches. See illustration.

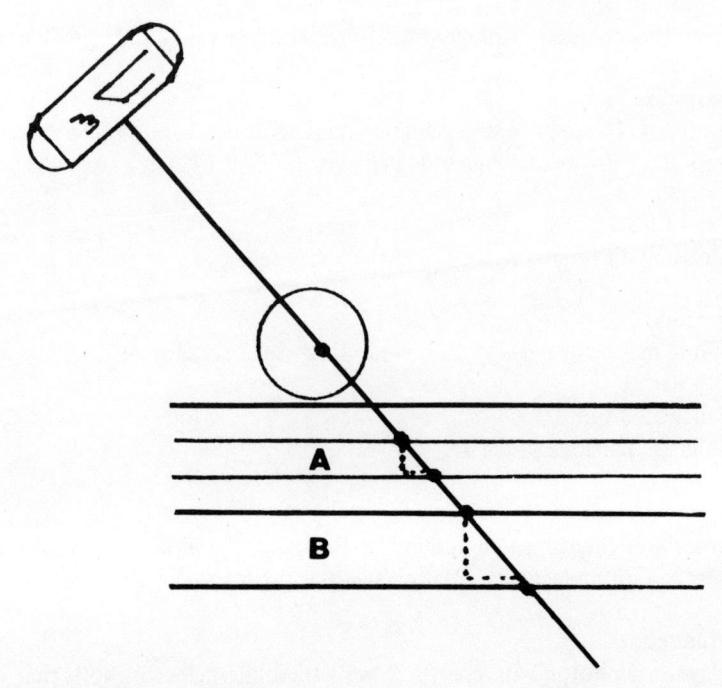

Parallax Film 'B' has a greater parallax than film 'A' because its thicker base separates the radiographic images on the dual film emulsion.

paramagnetic
A material, such as platinum, that is feebly attracted by a magnet.

parent
A radionuclide that upon disintegration produces a specific nuclide known as a "*daughter.*"

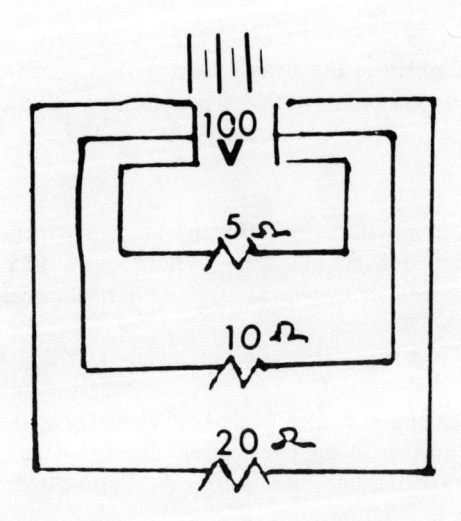

Parallel Circuit

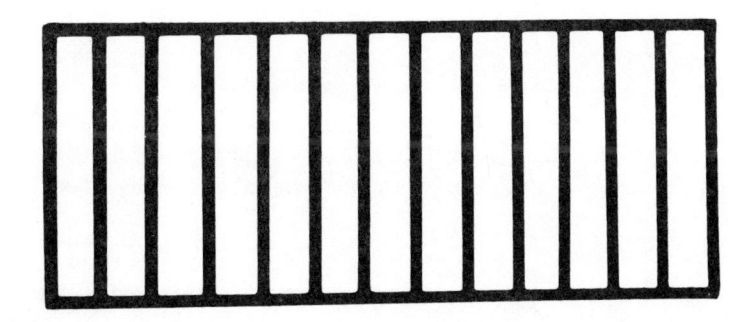

Parallel Grid

part-film distance
See *object-film distance.*

part-thickness
The measurement, usually in centimeters, of the part being examined.

passbox
A light-tight and x-ray-proof container built into the wall, with two interlocking doors arranged so that only one will open at a time. These boxes are conveniently placed between the x-ray rooms and the darkrooms.

peak kilovoltage (Kv.P.)
The maximum kilovoltage attained at any time in any sine wave cycle.

peak-to-peak
From a positive peak to a negative peak in an alternating quantity.

peak value
The maximum value of current, voltage, or power during the time interval under consideration. For a sine wave it is equal to 1.41 times the effective value.

P electron
An electron having an orbit in the P shell, which is the sixth shell of electrons surrounding the atomic nucleus, counting out from the nucleus.

penetration, radiographic
The transparency of the body images, bone, and tissue, that is controlled by Kv.P.

penetrometer
An aluminum step wedge, similar in appearance to elevated steps, that, when

placed over a film and exposed to x-ray, determines the quality or penetrating ability of an x-ray beam.

penumbra
The geometric unsharp appearance at the edge of a radiograph resulting from a large effective focal spot, a short target to film distance, and a long object to film distance. See illustration.

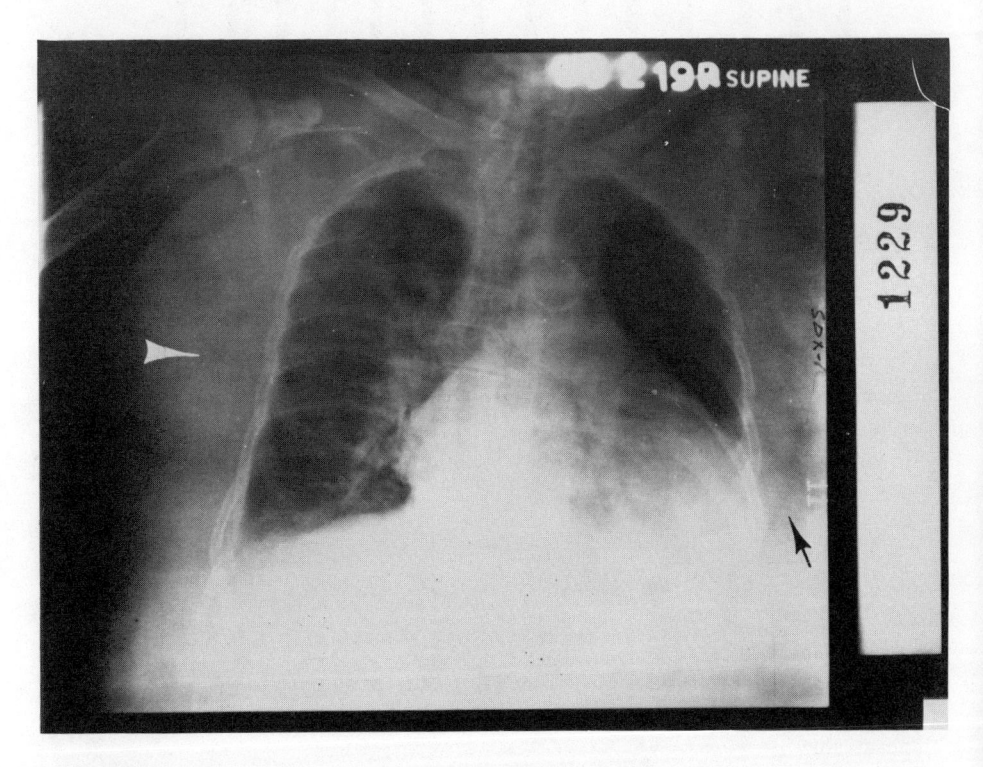

Penumbra   A portable radiograph demonstrating penumbra.

percent depth dose
That amount of radiation delivered at a certain depth in tissue, referred to as a percentage of the amount delivered to the skin, or in the air.

periodic table
A systematic chart on which elements can be arranged in a vertical and horizontal group table. The vertical group table shows elements with similar chemical properties while the horizontal group table contains elements with the same number of shells around the nucleus, but with different chemical properties.

permanent magnet
A piece of hard steel, alnico, or other magnetic material that has been strongly magnetized and retains its magnetism indefinitely.

permeability, magnetic
The ease with which a given material can be magnetized.

permissible dose
See *maximum permissible dose*.

persistence
The momentary storage, or retention, of some signal, or image, after the stimulus has been removed.

pH
Used in expressing both acidity and alkalinity on a scale with values ranging from 0 to 14 with seven representing neutrality, numbers less than seven increasing acidity, and numbers greater than seven increasing alkalinity.

phantom
An object that simulates the density of a body part used for radiographic demonstrations.

phase, electrical
The progress of wave structure of the alternating current with respect to the starting point of each cycle. Usually expressed in degrees, with 360 degrees representing one complete cycle.

phenidone
See *metol*.

phenomenon
An observation of fact or event of scientific nature.

phosphor
Any material having phosphorescent, fluorescent, or luminescent properties.

phosphorescence
A form of luminescence in which the emission of light continues more than 10^{-8} second after excitation by radiation having a shorter wavelength, such as by electrons, ultraviolet light, or x-rays. Also called *afterglow*.

phosphorus
Symbol *P*. A nonmetallic element. Atomic number is 15.

photocathode
A photosensitive surface that emits electrons when exposed to light or radiation. Used in television camera tubes, and other light-sensitive devices.

photoconductive material
A conducting material the conductance of which is a function of the amount of light incident upon it.

photoelectric effect
The effect of the photon from an irradiated body of matter after encountering a bound electron (electron closest to the nucleus) giving it kinetic energy. This effect is part of the process of the photoelectric interaction with true absorption.

photoelectric interaction with true absorption
When a body of matter is irradiated, some of the radiation (photons) will encounter bound electrons (electrons closest to the nucleus) and may dislodge the electron, giving it kinetic energy—called the photoelectric effect—and the emitted electron is then called a photoelectron. This type of interaction is desirable in the diagnostic region. See illustration.

photoelectron
This is the end result when a photon that has irradiated body matter encounters a bound electron (electron closest to the nucleus) and dislodges that electron.

photofluorography (photoradiography)
The process of recording the radiographic image with photographic technique. For example: a beam of radiation travels through the chest, falls on a special fluoroscopic screen at the end of a light-tight hood. The camera at the other end photographs the projected fluoroscopic image on a high speed photographic emulsion. The film sizes can vary and are: 16mm, 35mm, 70mm, 100mm, and 105mm.

photographic effect (PE)
The effect that radiation energy has to produce a latent image on the radiographic emulsion. This is expressed by:

$$PE = \frac{mA.S. \times Kv.P.^2}{F.F.D.^2}$$

photomultiplier tube
An electronic tube used to amplify the radiographic image of low intensity, that which appears on a fluororescent screen, and thus, the photomultiplier tube increases the image brightness hundreds of times.

PHOTON (X-RAY)

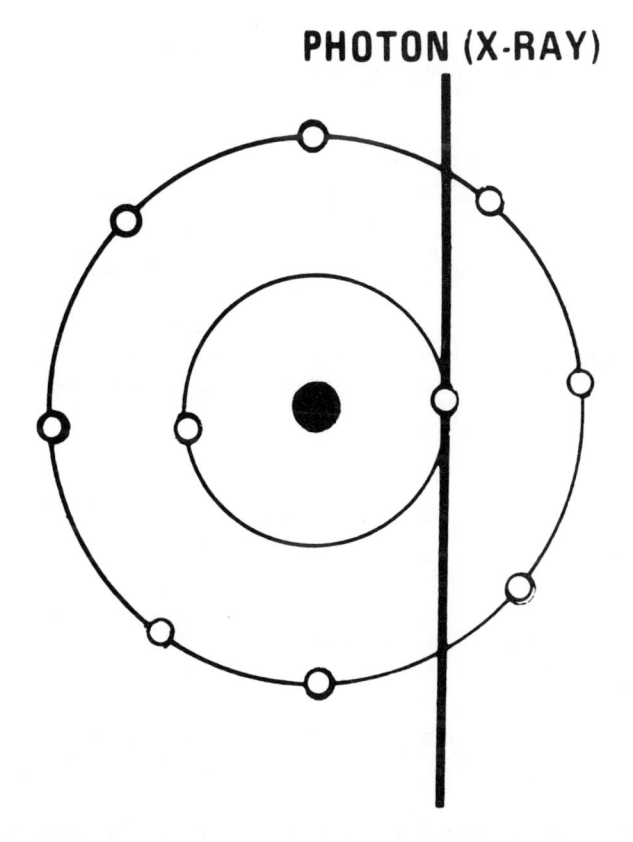

PHOTOELECTRIC EFFECT

Photoelectric Interaction with True Absorption

photovolt pH meter
Used to monitor pH to determine the effects of replenishment rates and check on exhaustion of developer.

photon
A quantum (bulk) of electromagnetic radiation. Electromagnetic radiation can be considered as photons of light, x-rays, gamma rays, or radio waves. Another term meaning x-rays.

photon theory of radiation
States that radiation is a shower of energy, heterogeneous in nature, traveling with the speed of light, and having no electrical charge. Sometimes called the *quantum theory*. Proton theory of radiation proclaimed by Dr. Albert Einstein.

photoscanner
Scintiscanner apparatus used to make a graphic recording of pulses derived from radioactivity of an isotope in an organism.

phototimer
A timer that automatically turns off an x-ray machine when the film has received the correct exposure as determined by an integrating photoelectric measuring system that monitors a fluorescent screen placed behind the film.

physicist
Member of the radiology staff who is chiefly responsible for equipment calibration, measurement and testing of radiograph systems and components, and so on.

physics
An exact science that deals with matter and energy and the interaction between them.

physiological effect
The effect that drugs or agents may have on living cells or tissues.

physiology
The study and function of various organs and structures of the body.

pi
The Greek letter π, used to designate the value 3.1416, which is approximately the ratio of the circumference of a circle to its diameter. A complete circle contains two π radians.

pick-up tube
The sensitive element in the television camera that converts a light image to an electrical signal.

piezoelectric crystals
Must possess an ionic charge that can interact with an applied electric field to produce a mechanical effect, for example, barium titanate, lead zirconate.

piezoelectric effect
Discovered by the Curies, 1880. Deformation of a crystal is achieved by application of a voltage across the faces of the crystal. The charge deforms the crystal and following the removal of the charge, the crystal surfaces vibrate harmonically at their high natural resonant frequency.

pig
A heavily shielded container, usually lead, used to store radioisotopes and radioactive materials.

pi lines
Plus density lines usually appear 3.14 inches from leading edge of the radiograph. Caused by a collection of residual gelatin and developer byproducts deposited in a long single line along a roller located in an automatic processor's developer transport rack.

pi mesons
Pions as they are often called, are intermediate in size between an electron and a proton; the mass of a pion is 273 times larger than that of an electron and one-sixth that of a proton.

pinhole camera
Designed to measure the dimensions of the focal spot of x-ray tubes.

pions
See *pi mesons*.

pitting, anode
Tiny depressions appear in the target due to overloading of the x-ray tube.

pixel, CT
Short term for picture element cell. The pixel is a representation of the volume element on the display.

Planck's quantum theory
The German physicist, Max Planck, formulated the following equation to represent the energy quantum:

quantum energy = a constant × a frequency.

plesiosette
A multiple screen cassette apparatus for separating films one millimeter apart to provide multiple tomography films with one exposure.

Plumbicon tube
One type of television pick-up tube that is very sensitive to light stimulation and is said to have a high resolution.

Plurigraph
The Picker tomographic system. Designed for pluridirectional and rectilinear tomography. It can also perform both as a flat bucky and erect routine studies.

pocket dosimeter
A fountain pen-shaped ionization chamber radiation monitor. The exposure may be read by a separate electrometer and is sensitive to exposures to .2R (200 milliroentgen).

point spread function
The image of a point object.

polarity, electrical
Direction of travel.

polarization
A displacement of bound charges in a dielectric material when placed in an electric field.

Polaroid Unit, radiographic
This mobile unit can process a radiographic image on photographic film emulsion within seconds after the x-ray is taken. Generally, it is used in the operating room for a rapid diagnosis.

pole
A region in a magnet that has polarity, such as the north pole or the south pole.

polyester
Base material used for film and screens comprised of dimethylterephalate (DMT) and ethylene glycol.

Polytome
Philips multidirectional tomographic unit.

positive charge
Having fewer electrons than normal, and hence, having the ability to attract electrons.

positive direction
Positive alternation or impulse of the sine wave.

positive electron
See *positron*.

positive ion
An atom having less electrons than normal, and therefore, having a positive charge.

positive terminal
The (+) terminal of a battery that has a deficiency of electrons. See *negative terminal*.

positron
A product of pair production that can join a free negative electron and disappears, giving rise to two photon with an energy of 0.51 million electron volts.

post evacuation film
A film of the large bowel made after the patient has evacuated the contrast medium.

potassium bromide
Restrains the action of the developer on the unexposed silver bromide grains without preventing the action of the developer on the exposed grains. Prevents fogging of the lighter areas of a radiograph.

potassium iodide
A highly sensitive negative material added to potassium bromide of x-ray film emulsion to increase the speed or sensitivity of the emulsion.

potential difference
Electrical pressure. It can be interchangeably used with electromotive force and voltage.

potential energy
Stored mechanical energy.

potential, electrical
Referring to voltage, or electromotive force (emf)

potentiometer
An instrument used for measuring voltage by balancing it against a known voltage.

Potter-Bucky diaphragm (bucky)
A bucky is a grid between the patient and the cassette which moves during the exposure and the purpose of which is to absorb scatter and secondary radiation that would otherwise impair the clarity of the image on the x-ray film. See *grid, radiographic.*

power consumed
See *power loss.*

power consumed (loss) **formula**
$I^2 \times R$ = watts.

power, electrical
The rate at which electric energy is taken from an electrical device, measured in watts—the product of the voltage times the amperage.

power factor
See *power formula.*

power formula
The work that electricity does in a circuit. E × I = watts
Electrical power is measured in units of watts.

power loss
The ratio of the power absorbed by the circuit in the form of heat. The power loss is proportional to the square of the current:

$$\text{power loss} = I^2 \text{ R watts}$$

power rule
The relationship between amperage and voltage in an electrical circuit. Power formula is:

power = amperage × voltage in watts.

power supply
A power line, generator, battery, or other source of power for electronic equipment.

prereading kilovoltmeter
The meter's function is to measure the applied difference of potential. Although voltage actually passes from the autotransformer to the primary winding of the high voltage transformer, this meter indicates the respective kilovoltage by stepping up the meter by a 1000. The meter is connected in parallel with the autotransformer.

primary, electrical
Primary winding or input voltage.

primary beam
See *central ray*.

primary radiation
Radiation arriving directly from its source without interaction with matter.

primary x-ray circuit
The primary or low voltage side of the x-ray circuit is divided by the high voltage and filament transformer's primary coils. The primary side consists of the following equipment: main switch, fuses, autotransformer, prereading kilovoltmeter, time, exposure switch, remote control switch, circuit breaker, filament ammeter, choke coil, and the filament primary transformer windings.

principal ray
See *central ray*.

proportional, directly
One quantity maintains the same ratio to another quantity upon which it depends.

proportional, inversely
One quantity varies in the opposite direction from another quantity on which it depends.

protective diagnostic tube housing
The housing is so designed that the leakage radiation measured at a distance of one meter from the source does not exceed 100 mr in one hour.

proton
Smallest measurable quantity of positive electricity. Positive particle of an atom.

P shell
The sixth layer of electrons about the nucleus of an atom, having electrons whose principal quantum number is 6.

Puck cutfilm changer
Rapid film changer utilizing punch card programming for angiography.

pulsating
Occurring in rhythmic beats, for example, the pulsating current in an x-ray tube.

pulsating direct current
Current that has been rectified from an alternating current source.

pulsation
See *alternation*.

pulse
A momentary, sharp change in current or voltage that is normally constant. A pulse is characterized by a rise and a decay, and has finite duration. Also called *impulse* or *alternation*.

pulses per second
The number of pulses per second in a sine wave. For an a.c. quantity, use cycles per second.

Pupin, Michael
Calcium tungstate fluorescent crystal screens were first used by Professor

Pupin in 1896. He worked with the screens that Thomas Edison sent to him.

Q electron
An electron having an orbit in the Q shell, which is the seventh shell of electrons surrounding the atomic nucleus, counting out from the nucleus.

Q shell
The seventh layer of electrons about the nucleus of an atom, having electrons characterized by the principal quantum number 7.

Quality Assurance (QA)
A performance of testing done at regular intervals, designed to monitor equipment to assure consistently good performance.

quality control
See *quality assurance*.

quality factor (QF)
A numeral factor that relates the biological damage of one type of radiation to an equivalent amount of x-radiation. For example, one rad of neutron radiation is 10 times biologically more damaging than one rad of x-rays.

quality, radiographic
Kilovoltage controls the quality of the primary beam. The quality, sometimes referred to as contrast, is the degree of gray tone that differentiates bony structure from tissue opacity.

quality, therapy
The filter (half value layer) that controls the quality of the primary beam of x-ray therapy units.

quanta
The fundamental unit of x-ray energy.

quantity of electricity
The amount of current flowing through a circuit at a given time.

quantity, radiographic
Milliampere-seconds control the quantity of the primary beam. The quantity, referred to as density, is the overall darkness of a radiograph.

quantum (plural, quanta)
The bulk of energy that can be associated with a given phenomenon. The quantum of electromagnetic radiation is the photon. See *photon*.

quantum noise
A random noise pattern. Created by insufficient absorption of the x-ray beam in the subject and/or input screen of the image intensifier.

quantum theory
For light or other radiation, the quantum is the photon, the energy of which is equal to the frequency of the radiation in cps. See *photon theory*.

rad
The standard unit of radiation absorbed dose.

radiant energy
The energy of electromagnetic radiation, such as radio waves, visible light, x-rays, and gamma rays.

radiation
Electromagnetic energy, such as light waves, sound waves, radio waves, x-rays, and heat rays, traveling through material or through space.

radiation burn
A burn caused by over exposure to radiant energy.

radiation counter
An instrument used for detecting or measuring nuclear radiation by counting the resultant ionizing events. Examples include Geiger counters and scintillation counters.

radiation equivalent man (rem)
A unit of ionizing radiation, equal to the amount that produces the same damage to man as one roentgen of high voltage x-rays.

radiation hazard
A health hazard arising from exposure to ionizing radiation.

radiation injury
The harmful effects are of two types, local and general.
Local: Exposures that affect the skin (erythema).
General: Exposures that affect blood forming organs (bone marrow and lymphatic tissues).

radiation monitor
An instrument that detects and measures radioactive particles on clothing and body.

radiation physics
Exact science dealing with radiation.

radiation therapy
The use of radiation in the treatment of disease.

radiation warning symbol
A standard symbol used on posters displayed in the locations where radiation hazards exist. The symbol consists of a magenta trefoil printed black on a yellow background. See illustration.

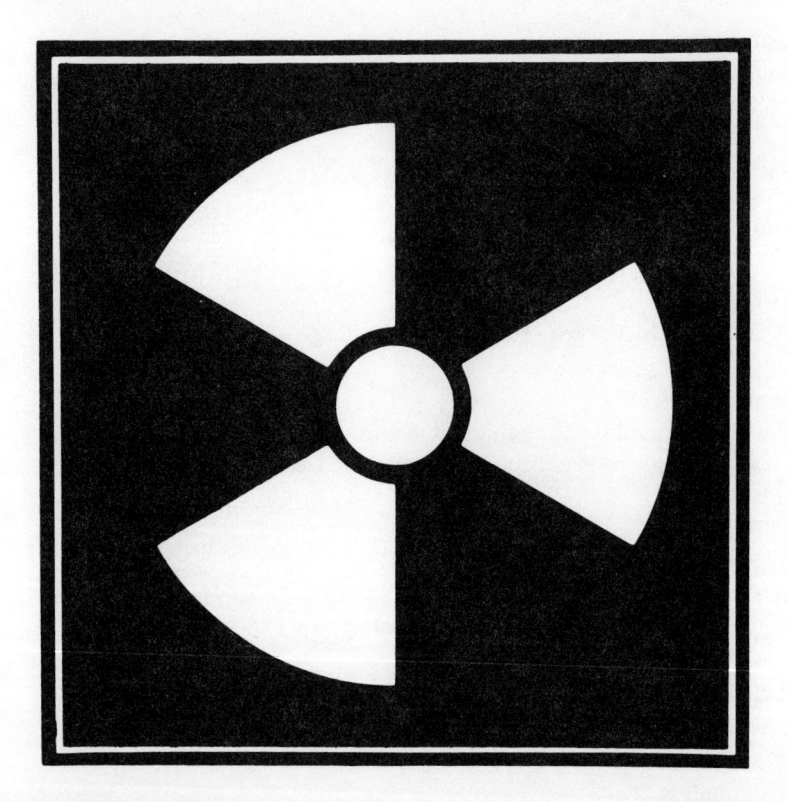

Radiation Warning Symbol

radiation window
A lead glass window that is transparent to light, permitting the operator to see the patient while protecting him or her from alpha, beta, gamma, and/or x-rays. This window is part of the control booth and is approximately five feet from the floor.

radioactive
Pertaining to or exhibiting radioactivity.

radioactive decay
The spontaneous transformation of a nuclide into one or more different nuclides. The process involves the emission from the nucleus of alpha particles, electrons, positrons, and gamma rays, the nuclear capture or ejection of orbital electrons, or fission. The rate of radioactive decay is expressed in terms of half-life.

radioactive element
An element that disintegrates spontaneously, giving off various rays and particles. Examples include promethium, radium, thorium, and uranium.

radioactive half-life
The time required for a particular radioisotope to decrease to half its initial value.

radioactive isotope
A chemical element that has been made radioactive. A radioactive isotope is produced by the irradiation of the nuclei of certain atoms.

radioactive source
Any quantity of radioactive material intended for use as a source of ionizing radiation.

radioactivity
A process in which certain nuclei undergo a spontaneous disintegration. Spontaneous nuclear disintegration of a property possessed by elements like radium, uranium, thorium, and their products. Alpha or beta particles and sometimes also gamma rays are emitted by disintegration of the nuclei of atoms. Also called *activity*.

radiobiology
That branch of biology that deals with the effects of radiation on living tissue.

radiocarbon
Carbon-14, a weak radioisotope used in biological and agricultural tracer studies. Half-life is 5,740 years.

radiocesium
Cesium-137, a radioisotope recovered from the waste of nuclear reactors. Useful for sterilizing food and as a substitute for radium in medical work. Half-life is 37 years.

radioelement
An element tagged with one or more radioisotopes.

radiograph
A permanent recording on film emulsion of a radiographic image produced when a beam of ionizing radiation passes through body matter.

radiographer
A person trained to practice the science of medical radiography.

radiographic contrast
See *contrast, radiographic*.

radiographic density
See *density, radiographic*.

radiographic magnification
See *magnification, radiographic*.

radiographic mottle
See *mottle, radiographic*.

radiographic quality
The characteristic summation of the various factors that combine to produce a radiograph that accurately images the anatomy under study.

radiography
The science of producing and/or recording radiographic images when a beam of ionizing radiation passes through body matter.

radioisotope
An artificially produced isotope that is radioactive. Many elements have as many as ten radioisotopes, produced in a cyclotron or by neutron bombardment in a nuclear reactor. Widely used in medicine, and other fields as radioactive tracers and as sources of ionizing radiation. Also called *radioactive isotope*.

radioisotope scanning
A procedure that maps the distribution of radiation within the body, from points outside the body.

radiologic technologist
See *radiographer*.

radiologist
A medical specialist skilled in the use of x-rays, gamma rays, and other penetrating ionizing radiations.

right-hand rule
Also called the motor rule. It states that if the thumb and first two fingers of the right hand are placed at right angles to each other, if the index finger represents the direction of the magnetic field, and the middle finger represents the direction of the electron current in the wire, then the thumb points in the direction that the wire will move.

ripple, electrical
The rectified current magnitude fluctuation that exists from peak to peak of a sine wave. There is a 100 percent rectified ripple in a single phase; a 13.5 percent ripple in the six pulse; and 3.5 percent ripple in the 12 pulse three phase. See illustration.

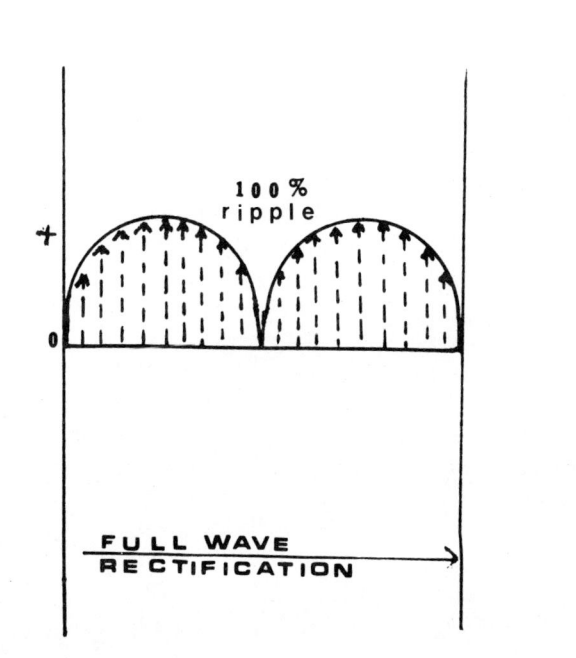

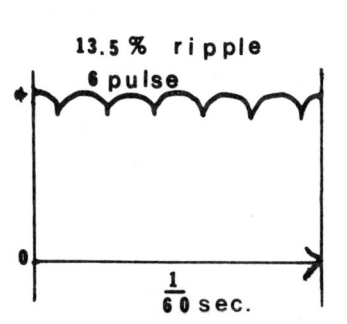

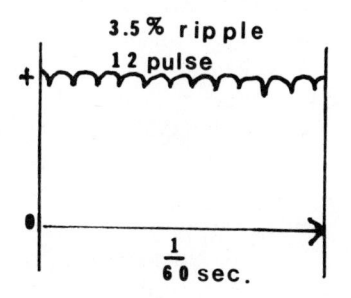

Ripple, Electrical

RMS value
See *root-mean-square value*.

roentgen (R)
The unit of quantity of X or gamma radiation. The international unit of exposure dose for x-rays and gamma rays. One roentgen of radiation will ionize dry air sufficiently to produce one electrostatic unit of electricity per 0.001293 gram of air.

roentgen equivalent man (rem)
See *radiation equivalent man.*

roentgen equivalent physical (rep)
A unit of ionizing radiation, equal to the amount that causes absorption, of 93 ergs of energy per gram of soft tissue. Also called *equivalent roentgen.*

roentgenogram
Deprecated term for *x-ray photograph.*

roentgenography
Photography by means of roentgen rays. Roentgenography and radiography are commonly used interchangeably as essentially synonymous terms.

roentgen ray
See *x-ray.*

Roentgen, Wilhelm C.
The discoverer of x-ray on November 8, 1895, by observing a Crookes vacuum tube operating at high voltage and a piece of barium platinocyanide lying a few feet away from the tube glow in the dark. Dr. Roentgen, a physicist, is known as the father of x-ray.

root-mean-square value (rms value)
The square root of the average of the squares of a series of related values. The effective value of an alternating current, corresponding to the direct-current value that will produce the same heating effect. For a sine wave, the rms value is 0.707 times the peak value. Unless otherwise specified, alternating quantities are assumed to be rms values. Also called *effective value.*

rotary converter
A device used chiefly to change direct current to alternating current to operate x-ray equipment from storage battery supply.

rotor
That portion of an induction motor that rotates during its operation, consisting of bars of copper arranged around a cylindrical soft iron core. It is sometimes called a squirrel cage motor because of its appearance.

rotating-anode motor
See *induction motor.*

rotating-anode tube
An x-ray tube in which the anode rotates continually during the exposure, therefore, having a fresh area for electrons to strike, allowing greater x-ray output and without melting the target of the anode. See illustration.

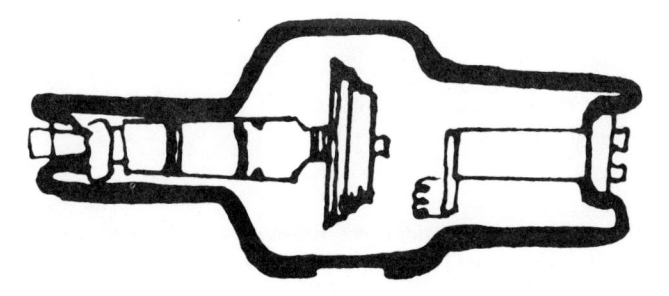

Rotating-Anode Tube

safelight
Special lighting used in the darkroom which permits film to be transferred from cassette to processor without fogging.

Sanchez-Perez
A rapid cassette charger allowing serialographic exposures to be made. Used for special procedure radiography.

saturable reactor
This new electrical device will replace the choke coil of modern radiographic equipment. The saturable reactor controls the current of the filament.

saturation current
The maximum possible current that can be obtained as the voltage applied to a device is increased.

saturation, tube
An x-ray tube functions at saturation, meaning the total electrons emitted from the filament are used during the exposure. In contrast, a valve tube functions below saturation (3Kv.), meaning the total electrons emitted from the valve tubes filament are not used during its operation.

saturation voltage
The minimum voltage needed to produce saturation current.

saturation point
The point beyond which an increase in one quantity produces no further increase in another quantity.

scan-a-screen
Ultraviolet scan device to detect the presence of dust, dirt, and defects of intensifying screens.

scan converter
A device that permits an image encoded into an electrical signal to be displayed on a television monitor.

scan, CT
The mechanical motion required to produce a CT image. In many machines a single scan can give rise to two images.

scan time, CT
The length of time that the patient receives the primary x-ray beam with the shutter open. The scan time is determined by selection of the scan speed.

scatter radiation
Radiation that has changed direction during its passage through a substance. It may also be increased in wavelength and called Compton scatter. See *Compton scatter*.

Schonander
Rapid film changer used in special procedure examinations. May be used in single or bi-plane angiographic examinations.

science
Subdivision of knowledge that is organized and classified.

scintillation
A flash of light (optical) produced in a phosphor crystal by ionizing a particle or photon.

scintillation counter
An apparatus that counts light emission (scintillation) caused by ionizing radiation acting on phosphor.

scintiscanner
An apparatus designed to map out the distribution of radioactivity in an organism.

-scopy (suffix)
Denotes the actual performance of an examination.

scout film
A survey film.

screen lag
A continued glow after the radiation has stopped.

screen mottle
See *mottle, screen.*

screen(s)
See *intensifying screens.*

secondary electron
An electron emitted as a result of bombardment of a material by an incident electron.

secondary radiation
Radiation produced by the action of primary radiation on matter. See illustration.

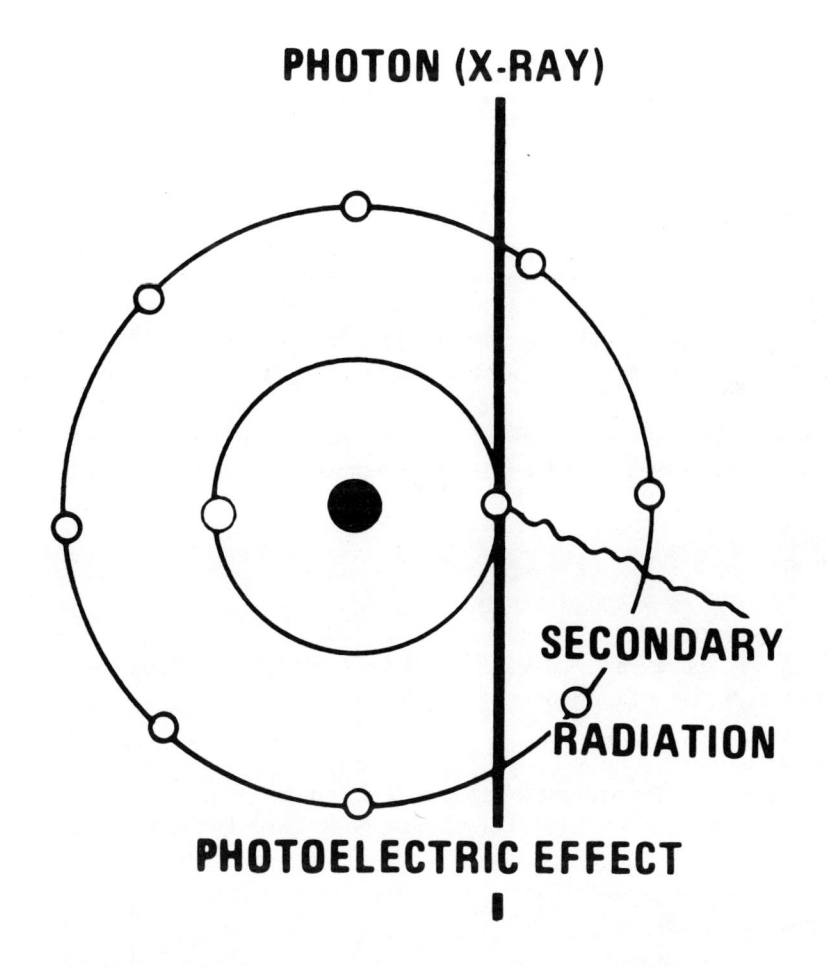

PHOTON (X-RAY)

SECONDARY RADIATION

PHOTOELECTRIC EFFECT

Secondary Radiation

secondary winding
Symbol *S*. A transformer winding that receives energy by electromagnetic induction from the primary winding. Also called *secondary*.

sectoring, ultrasound
See *compound scanning*.

seeds
See *radon seeds*.

selenium rectifier
An obsolete semiconductor solid-state rectifier which was used in the early 1960s for three-phase generator x-ray systems.

self-inductance
Inductance that produced an induced emf in the same circuit as a result of change in current flow.

self-induction
The production of the emf in a circuit by a varying current in that same circuit.

self-rectification
The negative alternation is directly applied to the anode of the x-ray tube, allowing electrons to flow from cathode to anode only during the positive alternation and stopping the electron flow during the negative alternation.

self-scattering
Scattering of radiation by the material that emits the radiation.

semi-
Prefix for half.

semiconductor
A material the resistivity of which is between that of insulators and conductors. Widely used in solid state devices.

semierect film
A radiograph taken with the x-ray table in the upright position approximately between 90° and 45°. For example, bowel obstruction abdominal films.

sensitivity, electrical
The electrical response that expresses the ability of a circuit or device to respond to an input quantity.

sensitivity, film
See *speed, film.*

sensitometer
Its principle operation is to make reproducible exposures on both sides of medical x-ray film for measuring and analyzing the performance of the processing system. Sensitometry is designed to determine the speed, gamma, and fog level for any standard x-ray film or cine film when used with a suitable densitometer.

sensitometry, radiographic
The relationship between the exposure factors and the processing conditions to the radiograph's response.

serial films
A series of radiographs that record progressive trace of the contrast media, for example, angiography.

serialogram
A series of radiographic exposures on a single film.

series circuit
Electrical circuit the component parts of which are aligned. Its characteristics are: amperage, constant; voltage, divides or varies; total resistance, the sum of all resistors in the circuit. See illustration.

service life
The length of time that a radiographic unit or other device will provide specified performance under specified conditions of use.

shadow shield
A gonad shield that can be attached to any beam restrictor. Designed for male or female use and can be stored out of the way when not in use.

shelf life
The time that elapses before an unused device becomes inoperative due to age or deterioration.

shell
A group of electrons that form part of the outer structure of an atom and have a common energy level.

shell-type transformer
Primary and secondary coils which are highly insulated from each other and wrapped around a common core.

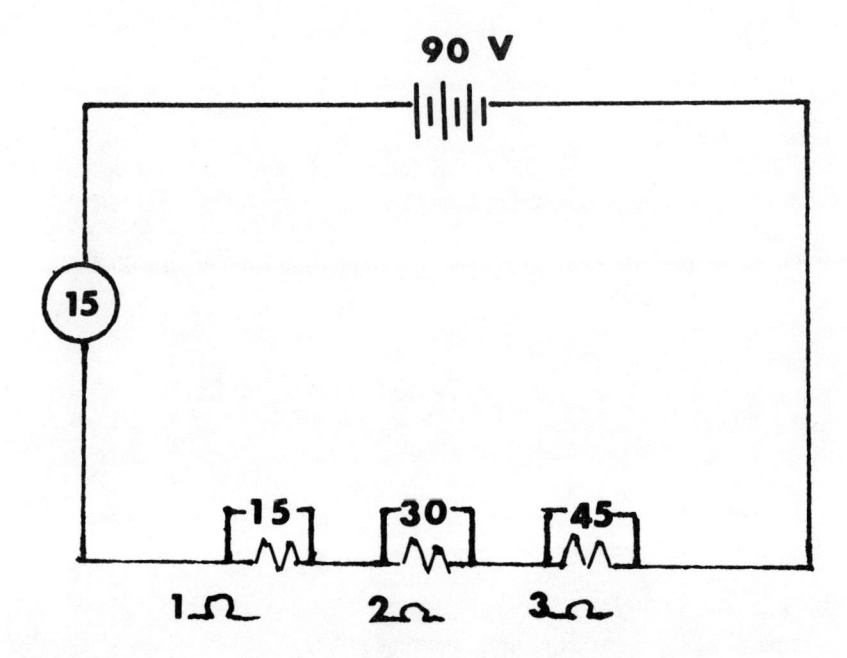

Series Circuit

shielding
Referring to protection from exposure. Lead aprons and gloves consisting of .5mm lead equivalent. The control panel for a diagnostic x-ray room should be lined with 1.5mm lead (1/16 inch thick) and should be seven feet high with an overlapping lead-glass window consisting of 1.5mm lead equivalent.

short circuit
A low resistance connection across a voltage source or between both sides of a circuit or line. Usually accidental and usually resulting in excessive current flow that may cause damage. Also called *short*.

short scale contrast
A radiograph having mainly light areas due to lower kilovoltages. A lower Kv.P. range produces five to eight shades of intermixed blacks and whites.

shoulder support
A mechanical device attached to the x-ray unit in order to support the patient's shoulders and body when the x-ray table is placed in a trendelenberg position.

shunt
To change direction.

shutters
Referring to moving lead coverings of a diaphragm, for example, the fluoroscopic screen shutters.

signal
Usually refers to an electric current varying at some frequency. Used to modulate another process, or is converted through a transducer into some form of energy to which the human senses can respond.

silicon rectifier
A popular semiconductor solid-state rectifier used for rectifying current of three-and single-phase generator x-ray systems.

silver
Symbol *Ag*. A precious metal element having better electric conductivity than copper.

silver bromides
X-ray film emulsion consisting of silver bromides and gelatin. The gelatin is dissolved in hot water under conditions of total darkness and silver nitrate and potassium bromide are added to make up silver bromide. When radiation strikes the emulsion, the silver (AG+) and bromides (BR-) join together to produce a latent image.

silver iodide
A halide that may be added to film emulsion to enhance sensitivity.

silver recovery
The method by which silver is reclaimed from exposed film and used fixer solution. This can be done during processing or through the stripping of discarded film.

simple molecule
An element that consists of all like atoms.

sine wave
A wave showing amplitude varying from instant to instant because of the plane of the magnetic field. The sine wave consists of frequencies and of wave lengths. One cycle is a full turn of the armature consisting of two impulses or alternations. The most commonly used alternating current is 60 cycle, having 60 complete cycles and 120 impulses. See illustration.

single pass scanning, ultrasound
A basic scanning motion that applies to the way in which the transducer is

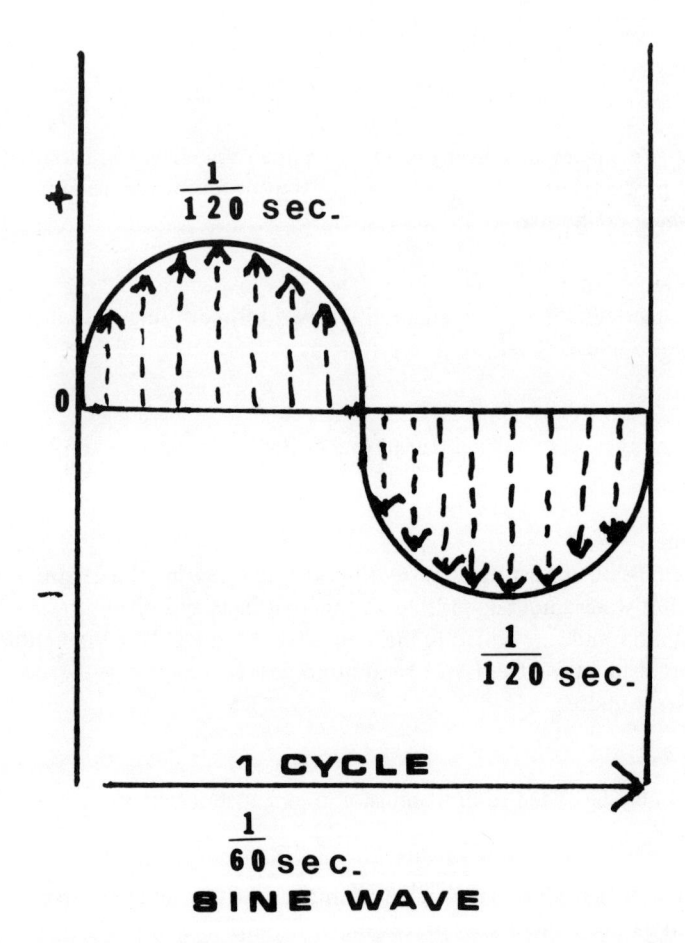

Sine Wave

moved across the patient to produce a scan. The transducer is moved across the patient in a smooth pass without arcing the transducer.

single-phase generator
A generator that produces an electrical current known as a sine wave. The armature of this generator rotates through a strong electromagnetic field 60 times per second, producing 60-cycle current.

single-pole double-throw (spdt)
A three-terminal switch or relay contact arrangement that connects one terminal to either of two other terminals.

Siregraph 2
The Siemens remote and table-side-controlled universal radiographic and fluoroscopic unit with an overhead x-ray tube.

Siremat
The Siemens fully automatic universal setup for diagnostic work employing magazine technique and an integrated processing machine.

Six-pulse three-phase generator
This generator system uses six solid state rectifiers working with three sine waves and resulting in a six-pulse ripple. See illustration.

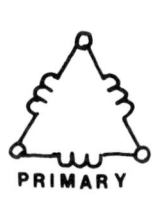

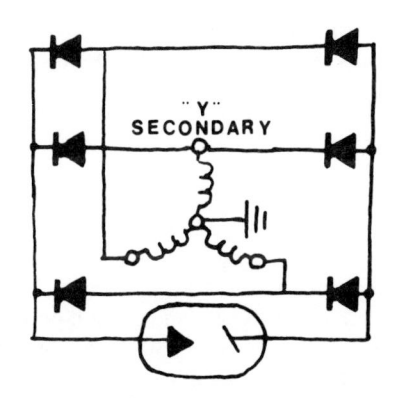

Six-Pulse Three-Phase Generator   The commonly-used wiring system operating with six rectifiers.

skiagraphy
A term used in the early days of x-rays, meaning radiography.

skin dose
The skin dose (surface dose) is the radiation delivered at the skin surface, and, with conventional x-ray therapy units, is the sum of the air dose at that point plus the backscatter.

skin reaction (erythema)
Skin becomes red from radiation or medication.

slice, CT
The cross section of the patient's body that is in the x-ray paths during a scan in which the x-ray source is rotated around the patient. The slice thickness is defined by the width of the x-ray beam.

slip rings
A conducting ring mounted at the end of the armature of the generator. The current leaves the generator through the slip rings to the external circuit.

sodium carbonate (accelerator)
One of the chemicals found in the developer that helps to swell the film emulsion making it easier for the developing agent to enter the emulsion.

sodium hydroxide
See *sodium carbonate*.

sodium sulfite (preservative)
In the developer, protects the hydroquinone and metol (developing agent) from oxidation. In the fixer, protects the sodium thiosulfate (fixing agent) from decomposition and helps clear the film.

sodium thiosulfate (fix)
Powdered fixer that clears the film by desolving unexposed, undeveloped silver bromides.

soft iron
Used in the manufacturing of cores for magnetic electrical devices because of its characteristics of high permeability and low retentivity.

soft-tissue film
A term used for an x-ray examination performed with relatively low voltage for the purpose of providing optimal contrast for evaluating soft-tissue structures. See *tissue technique*.

software, CT
Programs electrically preinstalled into the computer to provide all aspects of equipment operation.

soft x-ray
An x-ray having a comparatively long wavelength and poor penetrating power. This may be produced by lower Kv.P., light filtration, and targets of low atomic number.

solar energy
Energy from the sun.

solarization
A method of making a copy of a radiograph by exposing the unexposed film with the original film to light.

solenoid
An electrical device made up of a coiled helix carrying an electrical current. Solenoids are used radiographically for locks and Bucky trays.

solid pattern, ultrasound
Any structure recorded that gives the appearance of containing echoes.

solid-state diode rectifier
A silicon semiconductor used as a rectifier for x-ray equipment. There is a

stack of individual diodes connected in series, called modules, which stacking minimizes breakdowns. Solid-state diode rectifiers that were primarily used for three-phase are now used for modern single-phase x-ray equipment.

solid-state rectification
Used in place of the valve tubes to rectify the three-phase generating x-ray equipment.

sonics
The science dealing with sound.

sonogram
The scan produced by using ultrasonic waves; also called or referred to in many institutions as a *B-scan* or an *echo*. The proper term is sonogram but all are acceptable.

sonographer
One who activates the scanning device and manually or through automation produces a sonogram.

source-surface distance
The distance between the source or target and the surface.

south pole
The pole of a magnet at which magnetic lines of force enter.

space charge
The space charge refers to the effect of electrons emitted from the heated filament. See *thermionic emission*.

space charge compensator
A bank of resistors connected to the filament circuit that reduce the filament current to just the right amount as the Kv.P. increases to maintain constant milliamperage.

spark
An electrical discharge due to a sudden breakdown of air or some other dielectric material separating two terminals, accompanied by a momentary flash of light. Also called sparkover.

spark coil
See *induction coil*.

spark gap
A variable gap between points or spheres attached across a high voltage circuit in order to measure the approximate voltage.

spatial resolution, CT
The visual resolution obtainable of a matrixed scan image over the two dimensional area of the crt.

spatial filters, CT
An electronic system of introducing frequency filtering (into the video circuits) that has various attenuation curves and responses. The filtering is reputed to provide an accurate method of measuring the mean value of a specified image area, reducing noise, so large areas of small density can be visually resolved, and to enhance the display of anatomy and confirm the existence of certain types of artifacts.

specific gravity
The ratio of the density of any material to the density of water.

specific radiation
Same as characteristic radiation. See *characteristic radiation.*

spectrograph
A spectrometer that provides a permanent photographic record of a spectrum of radiation.

spectrometer
An instrument that disperses radiation into its component wavelengths.

spectrum
See *electromagnetic spectrum.*

speed factor
With intensifying screens, the speed factor is defined as the ratio of the exposure required without screens to that required to get the same degree of darkening of x-ray films. See *intensifying factor.*

speed, film
The term speed in radiography is used to refer to the relative amount of darkening produced on a film (with reference to film or screen characteristics) from a given amount of radiation, as compared to an exposure made with a different film or screen, as the case may be. Speed and sensitivity may be interchangeably used.

speed of light
Light travels 186,000 miles per second. All electromagnetic radiation travels at speed of light.

speed of x-rays
X-rays travel at the speed of light, 186,000 miles per second, or $3(10)^{10}$ centimeters per second in a vacuum.

sphere gap
A spark gap between two equal-diameter spherical terminals.

spinning top test
A flat metal top with a small hole through its edge. It is placed on the film and the technologist spins it rapidly during the exposure. The purpose of this test is to check the accuracy of the timer and whether all four valve tubes are functioning properly. Example: There are 120 impulses in a fully rectified unit x-ray circuit, and at 1/10 second, 12 dots should show on the film if the timer and valve tubes are functioning properly.

"split film" radiograph
A series of radiographs taken on a single film using a lead divider to cover the areas of the film not being exposed.

spot-film
A spot-film is an x-ray exposure, using a cassette, made during the course of a fluoroscopic examination.

stabilizer, filament
Its function is to correct instantaneously the tube current (milliamperage) when the line voltage drops because of demands for current elsewhere on the same line.

stainless steel
A chromium alloy steel having high corrosion resistance. Used in the manufacture of processing tanks.

standard
A reference used as a basis for comparison or calibration.

standard free air ionization chamber
See *Victoreen R-meter*.

Stanford and Wheatstone stereoscope
A floor model of a stereoscope made up of mirrors and prisms to display the radiographic image. It is not widely used because of its bulk and high cost. The hand-held binocular stereoscope may be substituted.

star winding
Also called "Y" winding. The configuration of the secondary coil for three-phase x-ray generators. See *delta winding*.

starter solution
The function of a starter solution (bromide, acetic acid, and water) is to enable fresh developer to perform as if a number of radiographs were already processed. Starter solution is only needed for automatic processor systems.

star test pattern
A tool designed to measure the effective focal spot size of x-ray tubes.

static electricity
See *electrostatics*.

static marks
Static marks resemble small streaks of lightning on a processed x-ray film, and result from static electricity when the film is removed from the wrapper paper or when films are separated from one another after being piled on top of one another.

stationary anode tube
An x-ray having a stationary anode. The anode consists of a block of copper in which is embedded a small tungsten button as the target.

stationary grid
One that does not move during the exposure. In 1913, Gustave Bucky built and used the first stationary grid, a flat, thin, rectangular device, approximately the same size as the film, placed between the patient and the film for the purpose of cleaning-up secondary radiation. The stationary grid was improved in 1920 by Dr. Hollis Potter, who conceived the idea of moving the grid, thus, improving the amount of clean-up and eliminating the lead strip pattern on the x-ray film.

stator
The portion of an induction motor that contains the stationary parts of the magnetic circuit and their associated windings.

steel
See *hard steel*.

stem radiation
X-rays given off from parts of the anode other than the target in an x-ray tube.

step-down transformer
Produces a lower voltage output than input by stepping down the input voltage. When stepping down voltage there is a step up on amperage because the power input is equal to the power output. The filament transformer of the x-ray circuit is a step-down transformer.

step-up transformer
Produces a higher voltage output than the input by stepping up the output voltage. When stepping up voltage, there is a step down in amperage because the power input is equal to the power output. The high-voltage transformer of the x-ray circuit is a step-up transformer.

step wedge
See *penetrometer*.

stereo-
A prefix used to designate a three-dimensional characteristic.

stereoradiography
A radiographic examination in which two films are obtained in rapid succession but with a predetermined difference in projection in order that the films permit visualization in three dimensions of an area in question. The total stereo shift distance is 1/10 of the target-film distance. More commonly referred to as a *stereoscopic examination*.

stereoscope
An instrument used to read stereoradiography. See *Stanford and Wheatstone stereoscope*.

stereoscopic examination
A radiographic examination that produces a three-dimensional visual image.

stop bath
A solution of water and acetic acid used between the developer and the fixer so as to stop the development of the film.

stratigraphy
See *body section radiography*.

stray radiation
Radiation that serves no useful purpose and is the sum of leakage and scatter.

streaky films
Usually caused by failure to agitate films in the developer, or in the fixer.

strontium-90
A radioisotope having a half-life of about 25 years. Also called radiostrontium.

sub-
A prefix meaning below.

subatomic
Particles smaller than atoms, such as electrons, protons, and neutrons.

subject unsharpness
See *absorption unsharpness*.

substance
Single kind of matter that has a definite, constant composition.

subtraction, film
In the field of radiology, the technique of superimposing two images. One is a negative, so that undesirable portions of the image are cancelled out. Makes fine detail contained in only one image more apparent.

sulfur
Found in film emulsion to improve sensitivity to radiation or light.

superficial therapy
A term used in radiation therapy for treatment devised to maximize the effect of treatment on the skin while sparing the underlying tissues.

supervoltage therapy radiation
A therapy unit operating at a potential of 4 mv or more.

supply voltage
The voltage obtained from a power supply for operation of a circuit.

suppressing, electrical
Refers to the sine wave, holding the inverse or negative alternation back by a diode tube. This term is used when referring to electrical rectification.

supra-
Prefix meaning above.

surface dose
See *skin dose*.

surge, electrical
A momentary large increase of the current or voltage in an electric circuit.

Sweet's eye
A radiographic method for localizing an opague foreign body in the eye, using a Keleket eye localizer.

switch
A manual or mechanical device for making or breaking, the connections in an electric circuit.

symbol
A letter or abbreviation used on diagrams or in equations to represent a quantity or to identify an object.

synchronization
The maintenance of one operation in step with another.

synchronizing pulse
A momentary pulse created in the television camera. Transmitted to the monitor in order to keep the two electron beams synchronized and scanning the same part of the picture at the same time.

synchronous
In step or in phase, as applied to two or more circuits.

synchronous motor
A synchronous machine that transforms a.c. electric power into mechanical power.

synchronous timer
A timer operated by a synchronous motor.

table, x-ray
A radiolucent top, on which the patient can be placed in the upright or horizontal position during an x-ray examination.

tank, processing
Metal tanks used to hold processing solutions. Constructed of stainless steel because it not only resists corrosion, but permits rapid equalization of temperature control. The outside walls of the tanks are insulated to prevent condensation of moisture and maintain temperature control.

taps
Taps are contacts coming off the autotransformer so that a specific amount of voltage can be applied to the primary of the high voltage transformer.

target
In an x-ray tube the target is the anode from which x-rays are emitted as a result of electron bombardment. See *focal spot*.

target angle
The target angle is the angle away from perpendicular at which the electron stream strikes the target.

target-film distance (TFD)
Same as focal-film distance (FFD), that is, the distance from the focal spot of the x-ray tube to the x-ray film.

target-skin distance (TSD)
The distance from the x-ray tube target (anode) to the skin of the patient where the x-ray beam enters his body.

technique
The components that comprise x-ray exposure for a given body part; mA, Kv.P., time.

tele-
Prefix meaning distance.

teleroentgenography
X-ray studies obtained with the tube at least six feet from the film, with the purpose of striving for parallel rays and minimizing distortion.

teletherapy
Term taken from the old "radium bomb" x-ray tube. The entire tube is shielded with lead except one small area where the radiation is emitted. The same methods are utilized today for cobalt therapy.

television camera
The pickup unit used to convert a scene into corresponding electric signals.

television field
That portion of the scanning cycle in which the picture is scanned once from upper left to lower right.

television frame
That portion of the scanning system in which the subject scene is completely scanned one time. In most cases, a television frame consists of two or more television fields, in some interlace pattern.

television lines
The horizontal lines used to create the television raster. Created by the path of the electron beams used to scan the pick-up and kinescope tubes.

television screen
The fluorescent screen of the picture tube in a television receiver.

temperature, effect on screen speed
If the room temperature increases, the speed of the screen decreases, but the two have a tendency to cancel each other. An alteration in technique under these conditions is not necessary.

temperature, electrical
Resistance in a circuit becomes greater as the electrical temperature increases.

theory
A proposed, but not a proven, explanation.

therapy tube
An x-ray tube designed for use in x-ray therapy. Such a tube operates at low milliamperage and higher kilovoltage than a diagnostic x-ray tube. The construction of a therapy tube is somewhat different from that of a diagnostic. The focal spot is much larger and a 45° angle stationary anode is used.

thermal radiation
Radiation in the form of heat, emitted by all bodies that are not at absolute zero in temperature. The wavelength range extends from the shortest ultraviolet through visible light to the longest infrared wavelengths. Also called *heat*.

thermionic emission
The ejection of electrons from the filament when heated. The amount of electrons boiled from the filament is determined by the selected milliamperage.

thermionic vacuum tube
Any electronic tube having a filament that emits electrons when heated—for example, x-ray tube, valve tube, photo tube, and others.

thermoelectron
Electrons emitted by heating metal as the filament of an x-ray tube.

thermograph
An instrument that senses, measures, and records the temperature of the atmosphere.

thermography
Photography that uses radiation in the long-wavelength emitted by objects at temperatures ranging from -170°F to over 300°F. Also called thermal photography.

Thomson scattering
See *coherent scattering*.

Thoraeus filter
A primary radiological filter of tin, combined with a secondary filter of copper to absorb the characteristic radiation of the tin, and a third filter of aluminum to absorb the characteristic radiation of the copper. In the range of 200 to 400 kilovolts such a filter hardens x-rays more efficiently than the usual combination of copper and aluminum.

Thoramat
The Siemens fully automatic setup for diagnostic chest work, employing a cut film magazine and a built-on processing machine.

thoriated tungsten filament
Any vacuum-tube filament consisting of tungsten mixed with a small quantity of thorium oxide to give improved electron efficiency.

three-phase circuit
A circuit energized by a.c. voltages that differ in phase by one-third of a cycle or 120°.

three-phase generator
A generator energized by three single-phase currents out phase (step) with each other by one-third of a cycle or 120°. See illustration.

threshold dose
The minimum radiation dose that will produce a detectable specified effect.

thumb rule
If the wire (conductor) is grasped in the left hand, pointing the thumb in the direction of the electron flow [(-) to (+)], the fingers encircling the wire will indicate the direction of the magnetic line around the electron flow.

thyratron
A gas-filled triode tube used for electronic timer and phototimers.

thyroid scan
A procedure that maps out the thyroid gland on x-ray film by the amount of uptake of 131I. The purpose of this scan is to record hot or cold nodules. Cold nodules are usually malignant and hot nodules are usually benign.

thyroid uptake
A means of diagnosing thyroid disease by measuring the amount of uptake of the gland (131I).

time
The point or period when something occurs.

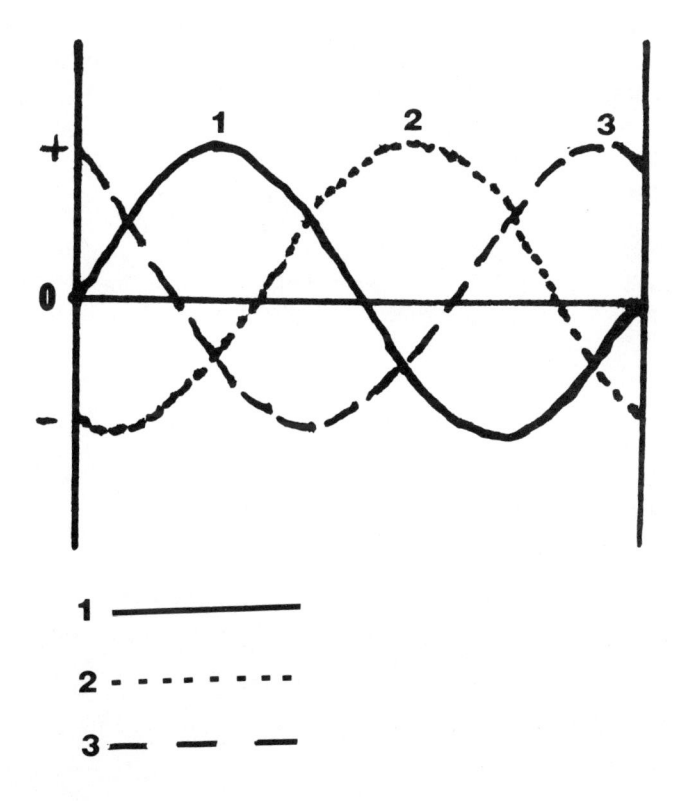

Three-Phase Generator

time exposure
The duration of radiation a radiographic film receives.

time gain compensation, time compensated gain
These terms are other names for the gain curve.

timer
An apparatus used to complete the electrical circuit of an x-ray machine so that x-rays will be produced for a limited period of time.

time sharing
A technique in which some component or system performs the same operation or function on many inputs. The different inputs are usually sequentially switched, so that the component periodically operates on each one of them.

time-temperature chart
A graph exemplified by the observation for optimum developing time for a given temperature of an x-ray film.

time-temperature developing manual
The universal time is three minutes and temperature, 68° F for developing most radiographic films. An increase or decrease of 15 seconds for each degree of change in temperature is recommended.

tissue dose
See *skin dose*.

tissue technique
A radiograph for tissue areas can be achieved by decreasing the original kilovoltage by ten percent and allowing all other factors to remain the same.

tolerance dose
Former term for *permissible dose*.

tomography
See *body section radiography*.

Tomolex
The Picker tomographic system with integrated tubestand which is an automated rectilinear device for horizontal tomography and radiography.

total filtration
Refers to the total filtration of the x-ray beam provided by both the inherent filtration and the added filtration.

tracer study
See *uptake*.

track
The path on a magnetic tape, or disk, that is converted into the magnetic reproduction of the input signal. If the track is scanned with the playback head, the original recording signal will be reproduced.

transducer
Any device which converts one form of energy to another. In diagnostic ultrasound, the transducer used can be of many frequencies and converts electrical to mechanical energy and mechanical to electrical energy.

transformer
Symbol T. An electrical device that can step up or down voltage from alternating current only. The component consists of two or more cells that are coupled together by magnetic induction. It is used to transfer electric energy from one or more circuits without change in frequency but usually with changed values of voltage and current. See illustration.

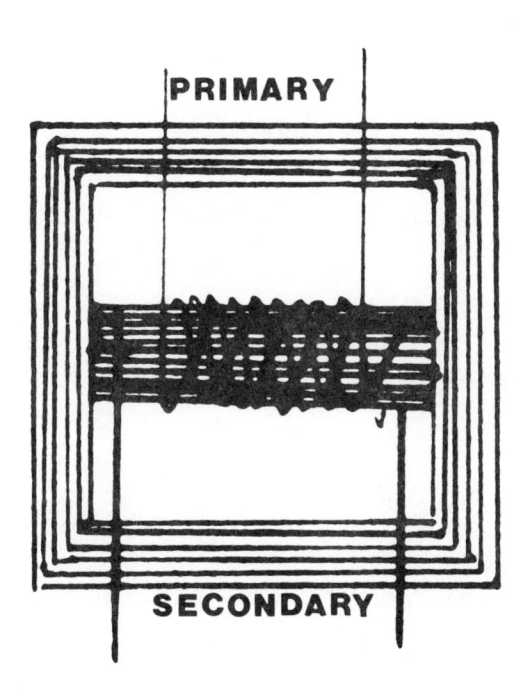

Transformer

transformer law
The voltage induced in the secondary coil is, to the voltage applied to the primary coil, as the number of turns in the secondary coil is to the number of turns in the primary coil.

transformer loss
The ratio of the power delivered by an ideal transformer to the power delivered by an actual transformer under specified conditions.

transformer losses
The three types of losses of electrical power in transformers and methods of controlling the resistance loss are as follows:

Copper loss. Because of the abundance of coil turns on the primary and secondary sides of the transformer, electrical power loss (resistance) can be minimized by a thicker cross-section of the copper.

Eddy current loss. Due to the intense heat of the soft iron core when the switch is closed, an electrical power loss can be minimized by the use of laminated silicon steel plates. Each plate is insulated from the next by a varnish, breaking up eddy current, minimizing power loss.

Hysteresis loss. Transformer operates from alternating current only and because the magnetic domains rearrange themselves every 1/120, this causes an electrical power loss. Such a loss can be reduced by using silicon steel cores. Power loss = $I^2 \times R$ = watts.

transformer oil
A high-quality insulating oil in which windings of large power transformers are sometimes immersed to provide sparkover.

translucent
Transmitting light but causing sufficient diffusion to eliminate perception of distinct images.

transparent
Capable of transmitting light so that objects or images can be seen as if there were no intervening material.

traverse, CT
In transplate-and-rotate CT machines, one complete linear movement of the gantry across the object being scanned.

trendelenberg position
A position in which the patient lies with head and upper body lower than hips.

triode tube
A three-electrode electron tube containing an anode, a cathode, and a control electrode. Some x-ray tubes are triodes.

Triphasix generator
A Picker x-ray system of three phase used in the United States in 1930. See *three-phase generator*.

tube cooling chart
See *anode cooling curve chart*.

tube current
Referring to the flow of electrons from cathode to anode of the x-ray tube and measured in milliamperes.

tube rating chart
See *x-ray tube rating chart*.

tube saturation
See *saturation, tube*.

tumor dose
Radiation dose given to a tumor. Measured in rads.

tungsten
Symbol *W*. A hard metallic element having a melting point of 3,370°C. Used for filaments and other electrodes of electron tubes. Atomic number is 74.

tunnel
See *cassette tunnel.*

turns, ratio
The ratio of the number of turns in a secondary winding of a transformer to the number of turns in the primary winding.

twelve-pulse three-phase generator
This generator system uses 12 solid-state rectifiers working with three sine waves, resulting in a 12-pulse ripple. See illustration.

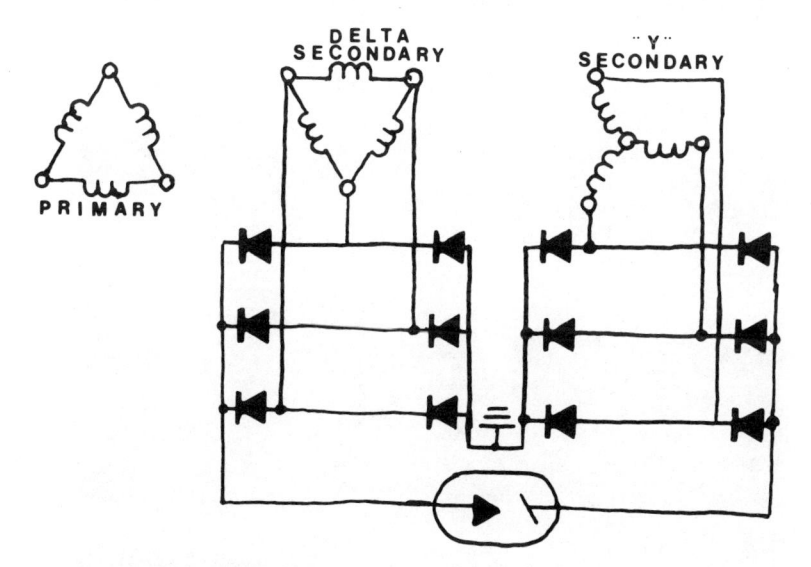

Twelve-Pulse Three-Phase Generator   The commonly-used wiring system operating with 12 rectifiers.

Ultracranio T
The Picker skull radiographic/tomographic system. The x-ray tube moves around the periphery of a sphere with the primary beam always pointing to the center.

ultrasonogram
A display of the ultrasonic wave recorded on photographic film.

ultrasound
Sound waves that are above 20,000 cycles per second or 20,000 Hertz (Hz)—beyond the range of human hearing.

umbra
It is the geometric sharpness of the objects that appears on a radiograph as opposed to its penumbra. See illustration.

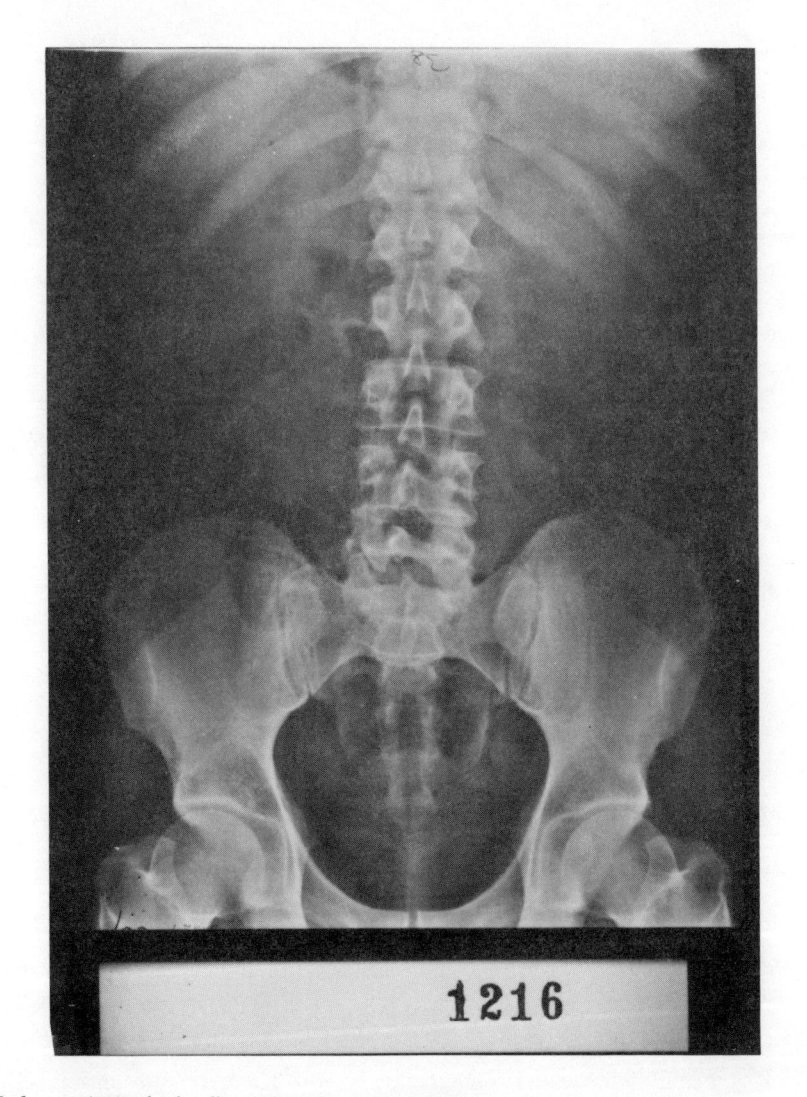

Umbra   A standard radiograph with true sharpness.

uni-
Prefix meaning one.

undirectional
Flowing in only one direction, such as direct current (d.c.).

undirectional current
A current that flows in one direction at all times.

unit
Smallest standard of measurement of size or weight.

unmodified scatter
See *coherent scattering*.

uptake
The quantity of radionuclides absorbed by tissue.

useful beam
The part of the primary radiation that passes through the aperture, cone, or other collimator used in radiology.

useful voltage
That half of the sine wave above the horizontal line. The half of the sine wave below the horizontal line is called *inverse voltage*.

vacuum
A space absolutely devoid of air, gas, or any matter, as between the cathode and anode of an x-ray tube.

vacuum tube
See *vacuum*.

valence
The outermost shell of an atom which determines the combining ability of that atom with other atoms.

valence bond
The bond formed between the electrons of two or more atoms.

valence electron
Electron that is gained, lost, or shared in a chemical reaction.

valence shell
The electrons that form the outermost shell of an atom.

valve tube
A valve tube is a vacuum tube of the diode type designed to permit the flow of electric current in only one direction within the tube. Valve tubes are used in the circuit to rectify the current. In modern valve tubes, the filament is thoriated to prolong its life. See *thoriated tungsten filament*. See illustration.

variable resistor
See *rheostat* and *choke coil*.

variac
See *autotransformer*.

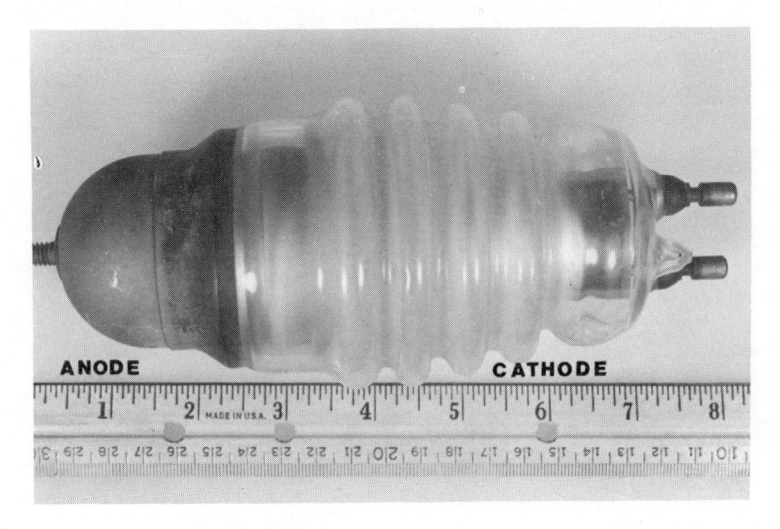

Valve Tube

Victoreen R-meter
Developed by H. Fricke and O. Glasser and incorporated by the Victoreen Instrument Company. It is used in calibrating the roentgen output of an x-ray therapy unit. One uses a thimble type ionization chamber which has been calibrated against a more precise instrument.

video
Pertaining to the picture signal of a television system.

video disk recorder
A type of magnetic recorder. Recording is done on concentric tracks of a rigid disk coated with magnetic material. It is basically a single frame device. However, frames may be recorded at normal television frame rates for short-duration dynamic motion recording.

video display unit
See *cathode ray tube*.

video tape recorder
A type of magnetic recorder. Recording is done as adjacent parallel tracks on a magnetically sensitive plastic tape. In playback, the image is displayed on a monitor, or receiver, with normal motion.

videx
The first x-ray beam collimator, manufactured by the Howdon Videx Corporation.

vidicon tube
One type of television pick-up tube, usually one inch in diameter and six inches long.

viewbox
See *illuminator*.

vignetting
A condition, created in an optical system, in which the intensity of illumination at the edge of the field is less than at the center.

villard
A full wave rectification system using charged condensers developed from a 100 Kv. transformer to 200 Kv. for therapy tubes. This is now obsolete.

visibility of detail
The optical sharpness of a radiograph.

visual acuity
The ability of the eye to resolve adjacent objects. Usually expressed as an angle.

Volta effect
See *constant potential*.

volt
See *voltage*.

voltage
Symbol E. The unit of electrical pressure, potential difference, or electromotive force. One volt will send a current of one ampere through a resistance of one ohm.

voltage compensator
See *line voltage compensator* and *automatic line voltage compensator*.

voltage drop
The voltage drop across a component or conductor by the flow of current through the resistance. The voltage drop across a resistor is usually called an IR drop, while that in a conductor is usually called a resistance drop.

voltage regulator
A device that maintains the voltage of a generator or other voltage source within required limits despite variations in input voltage. Also called *automatic voltage regulator* or *line voltage compensator*.

voltammeter
An instrument that may be used either as a voltmeter or ammeter.

voltmeter
An instrument for measuring voltage. Its scale may be calibrated in volts or related smaller or larger units. The E voltmeter is wired in parallel to the related circuit.

Voluntary Effort
Combined effort of the American Hospital Association, the American Medical Association, and others to reduce hospital expenditures.

voxel
Volume element of the reconstructed matrix. The computed attenuation coefficients correspond to the absorption in this volume which is dependent on slice width as well as matrix size. The term *pixel* may be used to describe a volume element as well as matrix size.

wash, processing
A part of film processing where the film is placed in running water after it has been fixed and before it goes into the dryer.

water path scanning, ultrasound
The type of scanning that utilizes a path of water between the transducer and the object to be scanned.

watt
The unit of electric power. The power in watts is equal to volts multiplied by amperes.

wattmeter
A meter that measures electric power in watts.

watt-second
The amount of electrical energy corresponding to one watt acting for one second. One watt-second is equal to one joule.

waveform
The shape of a wave, as obtained by plotting a characteristic of the wave with relation to time.

wavelength
The distance from any point on a wave to the identical point on an adjacent wave.

wave theory of x-rays
See *Maxwell Theory of Radiation*.

well counter
A counter used for measuring samples of very low radioactive materials.

"wet" reading
Wet reading is a term for viewing an x-ray part way through the darkroom processing, such as, during fixation or washing, in an attempt to expedite obtaining the x-ray information. This system was used before automatic processing systems used today.

wetting agent
Before placing the processed film in the dryer, it is recommended that a wetting agent, such as household liquid detergent, be used. This process reduces the drying time about 50 percent.

Wheatstone stereoscope
See *Stanford and Wheatstone stereoscope*.

white hot
See *incandescence*.

white radiation
Same as general or brems radiation which constitutes 90 percent of emitted radiation in the diagnostic range. The remaining 10 percent consists of characteristic radiation.

winding
One or more turns of wire forming a continuous coil for a transformer, relay, or other electric device.

wire
An insulated metallic conductor having solid, or stranded construction, designed to carry current in an electric circuit.

Wisconsin kV.p. test cassette
Used to provide a simple accurate check of kV.p.

Wisconsin timing and mA.s. test tool
This tool can be used to check the timers and the consistency of mA. stations of all x-ray units.

work
Force acting on a body over a given distance.
Formula: Work = force × distance.

Wratten 6B filter
The required filter for the darkroom lights with which most x-ray films can be handled safely without fog occurring. See *GBX filter*.

Xerg
See *electron radiography*.

xeroradiography
A form of radiography performed without use of x-ray film or fluorescent screens. A selenium-coated metal surface is substituted for x-ray film and after exposure to x-rays is dusted with calcium carbonate.

X-omat
Kodak's trade name for their automatic processing systems. Some types of x-omats are:
- Model M8—90 sec. processing—monitors ten functions and alerts operator to problems;
- Model M6AN—90 sec. processing;
- Model M7B—150 sec. processing—cold water;
- Model SP—2 min., 30 sec. processing or 3 min., 20 sec.

x-radiation
See *x-rays*.

x-ray beam
A stream of radiation produced when negative electrons bombard a positive anode of the x-ray tube. See *central ray*.

x-ray exposure fog
Fogging due to exposure to x-ray or radioactive sources.

x-ray generator
Referring to the step up transformer of the x-ray circuit.

x-ray pinhole camera
See *pinhole camera*.

x-rays (roentgen rays)
X-rays are a form of the electromagnetic spectrum, possessing the speed of light. The wavelength of x-rays is extremely small, in some cases within

the dimensions of atoms, and x-rays are capable of passing through materials that are opaque to ordinary light.

x-ray spectra
See *x-ray spectrum*.

x-ray spectrum
The wide range of x-ray and gamma wavelengths extending from one angstrom to milliangstroms and less, actually with no lower limits. The useful diagnostic range of the x-ray spectrum extends from 0.1 to 0.5 angstroms.

x-ray therapy
The treatment of disease using x-rays.

x-ray tube
A vacuum tube used to produce x-rays. The three essential parts are cathode, anode, and glass envelope. See *stationary anode tube* and *rotating anode tube*.

x-ray tube rating chart
This chart is a predetermined rating of how much Kv.P. and mA. can be impressed on a given target for what length of time. See illustration.

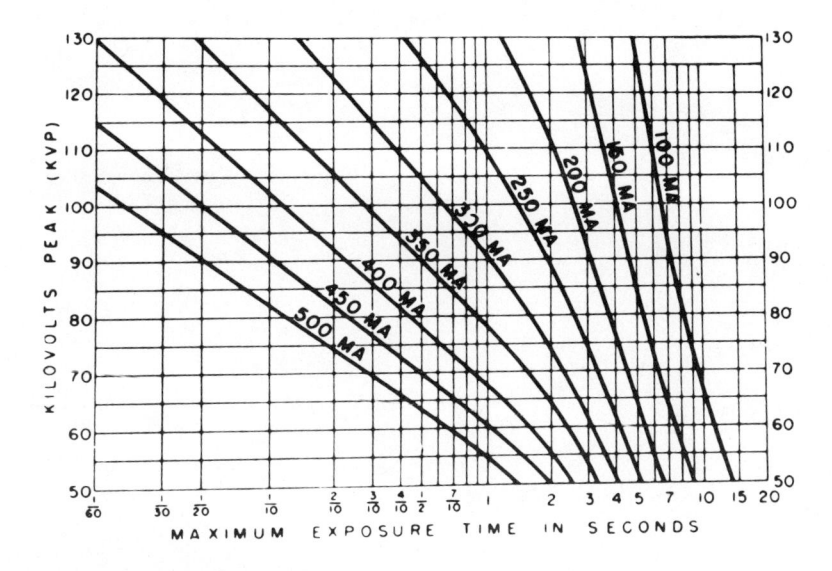

X-ray Tube Rating Chart

"Y" winding
See *star winding*.

zero potential
No voltage is flowing, electricity has stopped.

zinc cadmium sulfide
The phosphor used for fluoroscopic screens which emits green light which the eyes are most sensitive to at low intensity of the fluorescent light. The screen is backed with lead glass to protect the operator of the fluoroscopy examination.

zoom lens
A type of photographic, or television, camera objective having a variable focal length. This permits different magnifications to be obtained without moving the camera or subject.

ABBREVIATIONS

Å
Abbreviation for *angstrom*.

A.A.P.M.
American Association of Physicists in Medicine.

A.B.R.
The American Board of Radiology.

a.c.
Abbreviation for *alternating current*.

A.C.R.
The American College of Radiology.

A.C.T.R.
The American Club of Therapeutic Radiologists.

A.E.C.
Atomic Energy Commission.

Ag
Chemical symbol for *silver*.

A.H.R.A.
American Hospital Radiology Administrators, Inc.

A.I.P.
American Instititute of Physics.

A.I.U.M.
American Institute of Ultrasound in Medicine.

Al
Chemical symbol for *aluminum*.

A.M.A.
American Medical Association.

amp
Abbreviation for *ampere*.

amu
Abbreviation for *atomic mass unit*.

A.R.D.M.S.
American Registry of Diagnostic Medical Sonographers.

A.R.R.S.
The American Roentgen Ray Society.

A.R.R.T.
The American Registry of Radiologic Technologists.

A.S.R.T.
The American Society of Radiologic Technologists.

A.U.R.
Association of University Radiologists.

A.U.R.T.
Association of University Radiologic Technologists.

Ba
Chemical symbol for *barium*.

B.R.H.
Bureau of Radiological Health.

B.T.U.
Abbreviation for *British Thermal Unit*.

c
Abbreviation for *capacitor; cathode; celsius; centigrade*.

CAHEA
Committee on Allied Health Education and Accreditation.

C.A.T.
Abbreviation for *computer assisted tomography*.

c.c.
Abbreviation for *cubic centimeter*.

Cd
Chemical symbol for *cadmium*.

CGS
Abbreviation for metric system known as *centimeter-gram-second*.

Ci
Abbreviation for *curie*.

cm
Abbreviation for *centimeter*.

Co
Chemical symbol for *cobalt*.

C.O.N.
Abbreviation for *Certificate of Need*.

cpm
Abbreviation for *cycles per minute*.

cps
Abbreviation for *cycles per second*.

CR
Abbreviation for *central ray*.

CRT
Abbreviation for *cathode ray tube*.

CT
Abbreviation for *computerized tomography*.

Cu
Chemical symbol for *copper*.

DAS
Abbreviation for *data acquisition system*.

DB (db)
Abbreviation for *decibel*.

d.c.
Abbreviation for *direct current*.

DE
Abbreviation for *dose equivalent*.

D-max
Abbreviation for *maximum density*.

d.p.s.t.
Abbreviation for *double-pole single throw*.

E
Symbol for *electric field strength* or *voltage*.

E.C.E.
Evidence of continuing education.

emf
Abbreviation for *electromotive force.*

emu
Abbreviation for *electromagnetic unit.*

esu
Abbreviation for *electrostatic unit.*

ev
Abbreviation for *electron-volt.*

F
Symbol for *filament* and *fuse.*
Abbreviation for *Fahrenheit.*

f
Symbol for *frequency.*
Abbreviation for *farad.*

F.D.A.
Food and Drug Administration.

F.F.D. (FFD)
Abbreviation for *focal-film distance.*

F.O.D. (FOD)
Abbreviation for *focus object distance.*

fps
Abbreviation for *feet per second.*

FS
Abbreviation for *focal spot.*

G
Symbol for *conductance, generator* and *grid.*

G-M counter
Abbreviation for *Geiger-Mueller counter.*

H
Chemical symbol for *hydrogen.*
Abbreviation for *Hounsfield units.*

H & D curve
Abbreviation for the *Hurter and Driffield photographic curve.*

H.E.W.
Department of Health, Education & Welfare.

HL
Abbreviation for *half-life.*

H.M.O.
Abbreviation for *health maintenance organization.*

H.S.A.
Abbreviation for *health systems agency.*

H.U.
Abbreviation for *heat unit.*

HVL
Abbreviation for *half-value layer.*

Hz
Abbreviation for *hertz.*

I
Symbol for *current*.

I.C.R.U.
International Commission on Radiation Units and Measurements.

IF
Abbreviation for *screen intensifying factor*.

J.C.A.H.
Joint Commission on Accreditation of Hospitals.

J.R.C.
Joint review committee.

J.R.C.E.R.T.
Joint Review Committee on Education in Radiologic Technology.

K
Symbol for *cathode* and *relay*. Abbreviation for *kilo*.

Ka
Abbreviation for *kiloampere*.

Kc
Abbreviation for *kilocycle* and *kilocurie*.

Kev
Abbreviation for *kilo-electron volts* or *1000 electron volts*.

Km
Abbreviation for *kilometer*.

KO
Abbreviation for *kilo-*.

Kohm
Abbreviation for *kilohm*.

Kv
Abbreviation for *kilovolt*.

Kv.A.
Abbreviation for *kilovolt-ampere*.

Kv.P.
Abbreviation for *kilovolts peak*.

Kw
Abbreviation for *kilowatt*.

L
Symbol for *coil* and *inductance*.

LC
Abbreviation for *inductance-capacitance*.

LD
Abbreviation for *lethal dose*.

L.E.T.
Abbreviation for *linear energy transfer*.

log
Abbreviation for *logarithm*.

M
Symbol for *mutual inductance*. Abbreviation for *mega-, micro-, micron,* and *meter*.

m
Abbreviation for *micro-, micron,* and *milli-*.

mA.
Abbreviation for *milliampere*.

mA.S.
Abbreviation for *milliampere-second*.

mc
Abbreviation for *millicurie*.

Mev
Abbreviation for *million electron volts*.

mf
Abbreviation for *microfarad*.

MKS
Abbreviation for metric system known as *meter-kilogram-second*.

mm
Abbreviation for *millimeter* and *micromicro-*.

Mo
Symbol for *molybdenum*.

MPD
Abbreviation for *maximum permissible dose*.

mr
Abbreviation for *milliroentgen*.

mrad
Abbreviation for *millirad*.

mrem
Abbreviation for *millirem*.

msec
Abbreviation for *millisecond*.

N
Symbol for *neutral number*.

NC
Abbreviation for *no connection*.

N.C.R.P.
National Council on Radiation Protection and Measurements.

N.R.C.
Nuclear Regulatory Commission.

O.F.D. (OFD)
Abbreviation for *object-film distance*.

P
Symbol for *primary winding*. Chemical symbol for *phosphorus*.

Pb
Chemical symbol for *lead*.

PE
Abbreviation for *photographic effect*.

QA
Abbreviation for *quality assurance*.

QC
Abbreviation for *quality control*.

QF
Abbreviation for *quality factor*.

R
Symbol for *resistance* and *resistor*. Abbreviation for *roentgen*.

Ra
Chemical symbol for *radium*.

rad
Abbreviation for *radiation absorbed dose*.

RBE
Abbreviation for *relative biological effectiveness*.

rem
Abbreviation for *roentgen equivalant (in) man*.

rep
Abbreviation for *roentgen equivalent physical*.

RMS
Abbreviation for *root-mean-square value*.

rpm
Abbreviation for *revolutions per minute*.

R.S.N.A.
Radiological Society of North America.

R.T. (N)
Certified radiologic technologist in nuclear medicine.

R.T. (R)
Certified radiologic technologist in diagnostic medicine.

R.T. (T)
Certified radiologic technologist in oncology.

S
Symbol for *secondary winding*.

sec.
Abbreviation for *seconds*.

S.S.D. (SSD)
Abbreviation for *source-surface distance*.

t
Symbol for *transformer*.

T.F.D. (TFD)
Abbreviation for *target-film distance*.

T.S.D. (TSD)
Abbreviation for *target-skin distance*.

v
Abbreviation for *volt*.

va
Abbreviation for *volt-ampere*.

vdu
Abbreviation for *video display unit*.

V.E.
Abbreviation for *voluntary effort*.

w
Abbreviation for *watt*.

W
Chemical symbol for *tungsten*.

X
Symbol for *reactance*.

XL
Symbol for *inductive reactance*.

Z
Symbol for *impedance*.

TERMINOLOGY OF RADIOGRAPHIC EXAMINATIONS (PROCEDURES)

amniography
The radiographic examination of the pregnant uterus after injection of a contrast medium.

angiocardiography
The radiographic examination of the heart and vessels after injection of a contrast medium.

angiography
The radiographic examination of the blood vessels after the injection of a contrast medium.

angioplasty
A combination radiographic and surgical procedure in which special balloon catheters are used to dilate stenosed vessels.

aortography
The radiographic examination of the aorta after injection of a contrast medium.

arteriography
The radiographic examination of the arteries after injection of a contrast medium.

arthrography
The radiographic examination of the bone joint spaces after injection of a contrast media or air. The knee is the most frequent site of investigation.

balloon dilatation
See *angioplasty*.

barium enema
The radiographic examination of the large bowel after the injection of a contrast medium, usually barium.

bronchography
The radiographic examination of the lungs and bronchial tree after injection of a contrast medium.

cardioangiography
The radiographic examination of the heart chambers after injection of a contrast medium.

cerebral angiography
The radiographic examination of the blood vessels of the brain after injection of a contrast medium.

cholangiography
The radiographic examination of the biliary tree after injection of a contrast medium.

cholecystography
The radiographic examination of the gallbladder after rendering an oral contrast medium approximately 12 hours before the examination is to be done.

choledochography
The radiographic examination of the hepatic and common bile ducts injected through a postoperative T-tube.

cineangiocardiography
The motion picture radiographic examination of the heart and vessels after injection of a contrast medium.

cisternography
The radiographic examination of the cisterns of the brain after the injection of a contrast medium.

cystography
The radiographic examination of the urinary bladder after it has been filled with a contrast medium.

dacryocystography
The radiographic examination of the lacrimal ducts and glands after injection of a contrast medium.

diskography (discography)
The radiographic examination of the intervertebral disc after injection of a contrast medium.

double contrast study
A radiographic examination in which both a contrast medium and air are used simultaneously (or in succession in certain instances) for the purpose of outlining soft-tissue structures within the body.

embolization
A combination radiographic and surgical procedure using angiographic techniques to deposit glue or other embolic material into the area for treatment.

encephalography
The radiographic examination of the brain after filling the ventricles with a contrast medium.

esophagraphy
The radiographic examination of the esophagus after drinking a barium mixture.

femoral arteriography
The radiographic examination of the femoral arteries after injection of a contrast medium.

fetography
The radiographic examination of the fetus within the uterus.

fistulography
The radiographic examination of a fistula or sinus after the insertion of a cannula or catheter and injection of contrast medium.

gastrointestinal series
The radiographic examination of the upper alimentary tract after ingestion of a contrast medium, usually barium.

glandulography
The radiographic examination of the glandular structures after injection of a contrast medium.

gynecography
The radiographic examination of the female reproductive system after injection of air.

hepatosplenography
The radiographic examination of the liver and spleen after injection of a contrast medium.

historadiography
Radiographic examination using a special enlarging technique so as to magnify the recorded image.

hysterography
The radiographic examination of the uterus after the injection of a contrast medium.

hysterosalpingography
The radiographic examination of the female reproductive system after injection of a contrast medium.

intravenous pyelography
The radiographic examination of the urinary system after injection of a contrast medium.

intravenous urography
The radiographic examination of the urinary system after injection of a contrast medium.

kymography
Radiographic examination that records the involuntary movements of viscera such as the heart, the stomach, and the diaphragm.

laminagraphy
A radiographic examination of thin layers of the body tissue at any given depth by using an x-ray apparatus called a body-section unit.

laryngography
The radiographic examination of the larynx using a contrast medium.

lienography
The radiographic examination of the spleen after injection of a contrast medium.

lymphangiography
The radiographic examination of the lymphatic system after injection of a contrast medium.

mammography
The radiographic examination of breast using a special exposure technique and a special radiographic film or apparatus.

mesenteric arteriography
The radiographic examination of the mesenteric vessels after injection of a contrast medium.

metrosalpingography
The radiographic examination of the female reproductive system after injection of a contrast medium.

metrotubography
The radiographic examination of the female reproductive system after injection of a contrast medium.

microradiography
See *historadiography*.

myelography
The radiographic examination of the subarchnoid space around the spinal cord after injection of a contrast medium.

nephrography
The radiographic examination of the urinary tract after injection of a contrast medium.

nephrostomy
The radiographic (fluoroscopic) procedure performed to facilitate drainage of an obstructed kidney by the percutaneous insertion of a catheter that is fastened to the skin. This procedure may also use ultrasound.

nephrotomography
A body-section radiographic examination of the kidneys after injection of a contrast medium.

ordography
The radiographic examination of the thin layer of the body tissue at any given depth by using an x-ray apparatus called a body-section unit.

orthodiagraphy
Radiographic examination that maps out the bone or organ of interest.

pelvimetry
A radiographic examination of the unborn fetal head and outlet of the mother's pelvis for birth passage.

pharyngoesophagraphy
The radiographic examination of the pharynx and esophagus after injection of a contrast medium.

phlebography
The radiographic examination of the veins after injection of a contrast medium.

placentography
The radiographic examination of the gravid uterus for localization of the placenta.

planigraphy
A radiographic examination of thin layers of the body tissue at any given depth by using an x-ray apparatus called a body-section unit.

pneumoarthrography
The radiographic examination of the bony joint spaces after injection of a contrast medium or air.

pneumocystography
The radiographic examination of the urinary bladder after injection of gas or air.

pneumoencephalography
The radiographic examination of the skull after the injection of air or gas into the ventricles.

pneumoperitoneography
The radiographic examination of the peritoneum and intra-abdominal organs after the injection of air.

portography
The radiographic examination of the portal system after injection of a contrast medium.

portosplenography
The radiographic examination of the portal system or spleen after injection of a contrast medium.

portovenography
See *portosplenography*.

prostatography
The radiographic examination of the prostate gland.

pyelography
The radiographic examination of the urinary system after injection of a contrast medium.

renal arteriography
The radiographic examination of the blood vessels of the kidney after injection of a contrast medium.

retrograde urography
The radiographic examination of the urinary system after injection of a contrast medium through a catheter inserted into the ureters.

salpingography
The radiographic examination of the female reproductive system after injection of a contrast medium.

scanography
A special radiographic technique using a measuring tape device to measure the length of the femurs on a radiograph.

serialoangiocardiography
The radiographic examination of the various vascular systems with rapid serial x-ray exposures after injection of a contrast medium.

sialography
The radiographic examination of the salivary ducts and glands after injection of a contrast medium.

sinography
See *fistulography*.

small bowel series
The radiographic examination of the small bowel after ingestion of a contrast medium, usually barium.

splenoportography
The radiographic examination of the spleen and liver after injection of a contrast medium.

stereoradiography
See in general glossary.

stereotaxis
Surgical technique, in which radiography and/or fluoroscopy are used to place precisely probes or cannulas.

stratigraphy
A radiographic examination of thin layers of the body tissue at any given depth by using an x-ray apparatus called a body-section unit.

tautography
The radiographic examination of an angiographic procedure utilizing rapid serial equipment.

teleoentgenography
Any radiographic examination taken with a 72" target-film distance.

therapeutic embolization
See *embolization*.

thoracic aortography
The radiographic examination of the aorta in which a catheter has been passed through a peripheral artery and then injected with a contrast medium.

tomography
The radiographic examination of the thin layers of the body tissue at any given depth by using an x-ray apparatus called a body-section unit.

ultrasonography
A diagnostic procedure that employs the use of high-frequency sound waves.

ureterocystography
The radiographic examination of the ureters and urinary bladder after injection of a contrast medium.

ureterography
The radiographic examination of the ureters after injection of a contrast medium.

urethrocystography
The radiographic examination of the urethra and urinary bladder after injection of a contrast medium.

urethrography
The radiographic examination of the urethra during the injection of a contrast medium or during voiding.

urography
The radiographic examination of the urinary tract after injection of a contrast medium.

uterosalpingography
See *hysterosalpingography*.

vaginography
The radiographic examination of the structure of the vagina after injection of a contrast medium.

vasography
The radiographic examination of the vessels and lymphatic system after injection of a contrast medium.

venography
The radiographic examination of the venous structures after injection of a contrast medium.

ventriculography
The radiographic examination of the ventricles of the brain after injection of air or gas.

zonography
The radiographic examination using the principles of tomography to obtain thick body-section cuts by maintaining narrow ($10°$ or less) angles of tube movement.

ELECTRICAL SYMBOLS

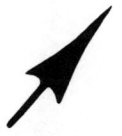

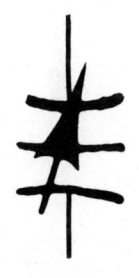

Adjustable

Adjustable capacitor

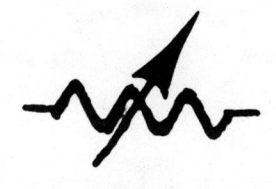

Adjustable resistor

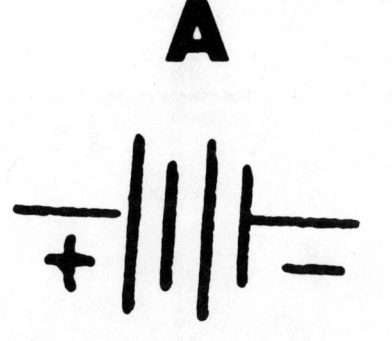

Ammeter

Battery

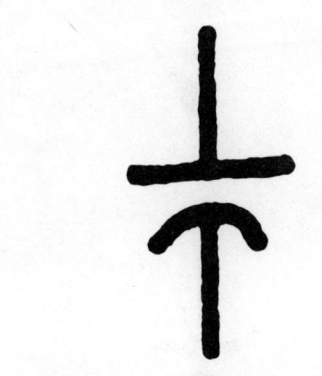

Capacitor

Circuit breaker

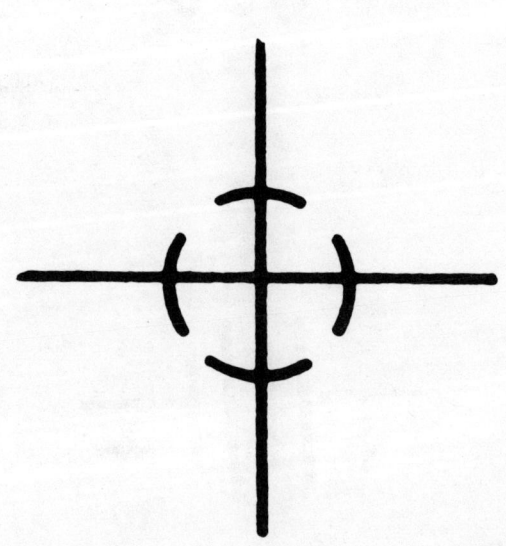

Crossed wire connected

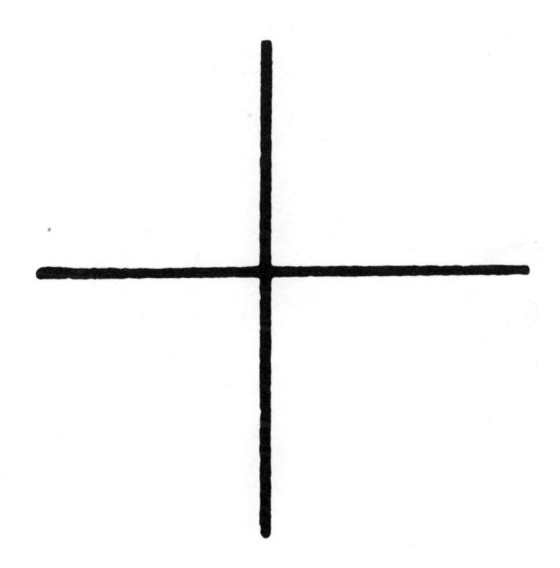

Crossed wire not connected

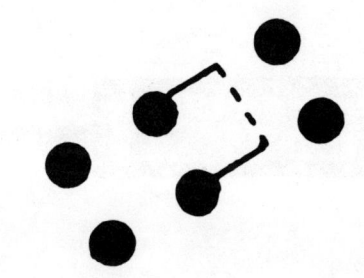

Double-blade single-throw

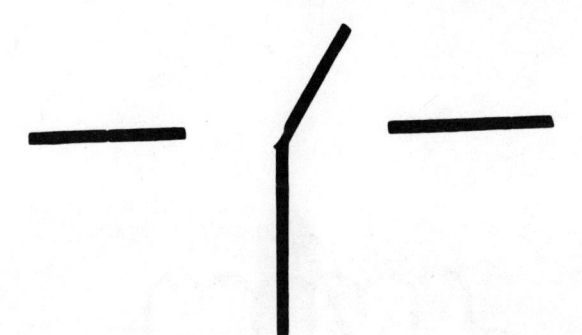

Double-throw switch

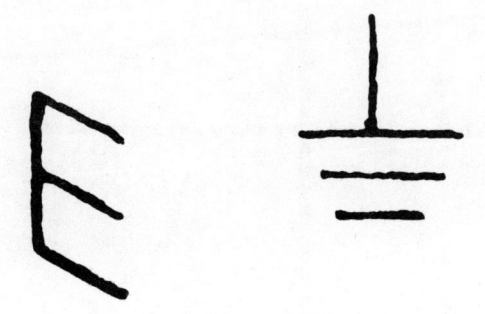

Earth or ground

Filament ammeter

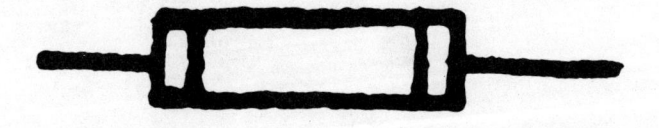

Fuse

Galvanometer

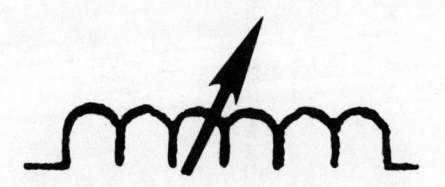

Inductor adjustable

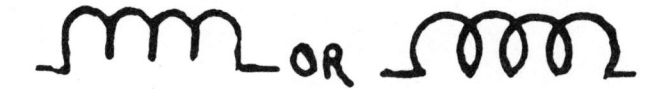

Inductor winding

PV

Pre-reading voltmeter

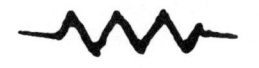

Resistor

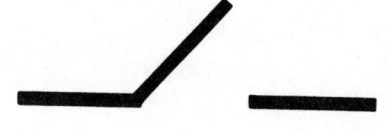

Switch

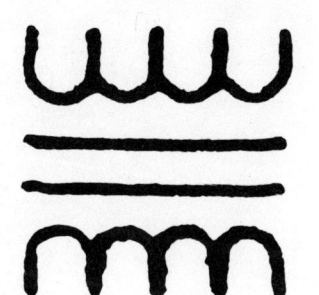

Transformer

V

Voltmeter

X-RAY CIRCUIT

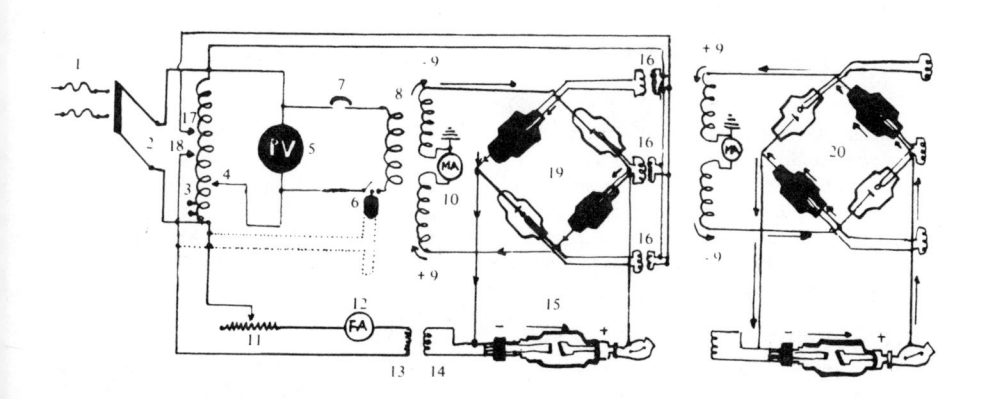

FUSES
1. Found at the incoming line to the X-ray room. Fuses are used to protect the X-ray equipment from electrical over-loading.

2. MAIN SWITCH
This double blade, single throw switch is located at the control panel.

3. LINE VOLTAGE COMPENSATOR
This adjusts the incoming line to the calibrated amount of the source voltage. This switch can either be controlled manually or automatically depending on the X-ray equipment manufacturer.

4. AUTOTRANSFORMER
This transformer is remotely controlled as the operator turns the Kv.P. dial at the control panel. The amount of voltage that is selected is then supplied to the primary side of the high voltage transformer (step-up).

5. PREREADING KILOVOLTMETER
This ac voltmeter, which is connected in parallel with the autotransformer, will correct any fluxuation of the main line between the autotransformer and the X-ray transformer primary.

6. X-RAY EXPOSURE SWITCH
This switch controls the length of time the X-ray exposure will last. There are four types of timers universally used today. They are: (a) synchronous timer, is accurate between 1/20 to 20 seconds. but cannot function below 1/20 sec. (b) motor-driven impulse timer, it functions at a high rate of speed; i.e., from 1/120 to 1/5 second time exposure. (c) electronic timer, operates between 1/30 to 20 seconds time exposure, (d) electronic impulse timer, functions accurately from 1/120 to 20 second time exposure.

7. CIRCUIT BREAKER
Along with the fuses (1), the circuit breaker is an additional protection against electrical overloading.

8. PRIMARY SIDE X-RAY TRANSFORMER
This is the input side of the high voltage transformer; it accepts the voltage selected at the autotransformer.

9. SECONDARY SIDE X-RAY TRANSFORMER
This is the multiplier of the primary side of the high voltage transformer; i.e., it steps up the primary voltage by the predetermined ratio of the transformer. If, for example, you have 100 volts applied to the primary and the transformer is a 1000: 1, the output voltage will be 100,000 or 100 Kv.P.

10. GROUNDED MILLIAMMETER
This grounded meter is connected in series with the secondary side of the X-ray transformer and measures the milliamperage of the X-ray tube. It is grounded at the highest point of voltage of the X-ray circuit.

11. CHOKE COIL OR SATURABLE REACTOR
This variable resistor operates between 3 to 5 amps and 4 to 15 volts; controls the filament current.

12. FILAMENT AMMETER
This meter is placed in series with the filament circuit and measures the filament current.

13. THE PRIMARY SIDE OF FILAMENT TRANSFORMER
This is the input side of the step down transformer which accepts the voltage that has been adjusted the choke coil.

14. SECONDARY SIDE FILAMENT TRANSFORMER
These winding step down the voltage of the primary side (13).

15. X-RAY TUBE
(See general glossary).

16. VALVE TUBE TRANSFORMERS
This step down transformer supplies current to the valve or rectifying tubes.

17. VALVE TUBE CURRENT SUPPLY
The source of current which supplies electricity to the valve tube transformers (16).

18. FILAMENT CURRENT SUPPLY
The source of current which supplies electricity to filament circuit.
(No. 19 & 20 IS THE TRACE OF THE FULL WAVE RECTIFICATION SYSTEM FOR SINGLE PHASE GENERATORS.)

19. ONE HALF CYCLE OR ALTERNATION
(1/120 second) This half cycle starts from the over abundance of electrons (-) to the deficiency of electrons (+) (9). Follow the arrows as the current passes thru the black valve tube, thru the X-ray tube (15,) and back thru the black valve tube.

20. SECOND HALF OF COMPLETE CYCLE OR ALTERNATION
(1/120 second) The over abundance of electrons (-) has now traveled to opposite or the lower end of the secondary side of the X-ray transformer (9). Follow the arrow as the current now passes thru the black valve tube, thru the X-ray tube (15), and now back thru the last remaining valve tube.

WEIGHTS AND MEASURES

COMMON U.S. MEASURES
Linear
12 inches = 1 foot
3 feet = 1 yard
5½ yards (16½ feet) = 1 rod
40 rods (220 yards) = 1 furlong
8 furlongs (5,280 feet) = 1 mile
3 miles = 1 league
1.150 miles (approx.) = 1 nautical mile

Volume
4 gills = 1 pint = 28.875 cubic inches
2 pints = 1 quart = 57.75 cubic inches
4 quarts = 1 gallon = 231 cubic inches

Dry Measures
2 pints = 1 quart
8 quarts = 1 peck = 537.605 cubic inches
4 pecks = 1 bushel

Area
144 square inches = 1 square foot
9 square feet = 1 square yard
30¼ square yards = 1 square rod
160 square rods = 1 acre
640 acres = 1 square mile

Weight (Avoirdupois)
16 drams = 1 ounce
16 ounces = 1 pound
2,000 pounds = 1 ton

Troy Weight (Jewelry)
24 grains = 1 pennyweight
1 carat = 3.086 grains = 200 milligrams
20 pennyweights = 1 ounce
12 ounces = 1 pound

Other Units
1 barrel (liquid) = 31 to 42 gallons
1 board foot (lumber) = 12 × 12 × 1 inches
1 bolt (cloth) = 40 yards
1 cable = 720 feet
1 cord (firewood) = 128 cubic feet

1 cubit = 18 inches
1 decibel = Smallest change in loudness detectable by human ear
1 fathom = 6 feet
1 gross = 12 dozen = 144
1 hand = four inches
1 hogshead (liquid) = 2 barrels
1 magnum (bottle) = 2 quarts
1 parsec = 3.26 light years
1 pipe (liquid) = 2 hogsheads
1 quire (paper) = 25 sheets
1 ream (paper) = 500 sheets
1 stone = 14 pounds
1 watt = 1 ampere × 1 volt

ROMAN NUMERALS

I = 1	VI = 6	XX = 20	LXX = 70
II = 2	VII = 7	XXX = 30	LXXX = 80
III = 3	VIII = 8	XL = 40	XC = 90
IV = 4	IX = 9	L = 50	C = 100
V = 5	X = 10	LX = 60	

COMPUTATIONS

Circumference of a circle; multiply diameter by 3.1416.

Area of a circle; multiply square of diameter by .7854.

Diameter of a circle; multiply circumference by .31831.

Area of parallelogram; multiply base by altitude.

Area of a triangle; multiply base by ½ perpendicular height.

Area of a rectangle; multiply length by breadth.

Volume of a sphere; cube diameter and multiply by .5236.

Surface of a sphere; square diameter and multiply by 3.1416.

Volume of a cylinder; multiply the square of the radius of the base by 3.1416 and multiply by the height.

METRIC CONVERSION

The United States, which has been the only large country not on the metric system, is rapidly changing over. Thinking metric means meter instead of yard, roughly three kilometers to every two miles, thirty grams to the ounce, two pounds to the kilogram, liter instead of quart, two and a half acres to the hectare (see table for exact equivalents).

Metric cooking is based on measuring utensils marked in milliliters and deciliters (1dl = 100 ml).

Measuring spoons:
1 tablespoon = 15 milliliters
1 teaspoon = 5 milliliters
½ teaspoon = 2.5 milliliters
¼ teaspoon = 1.25 milliliters

TEMPERATURE

To convert Centigrade* into Fahrenheit: Multiply Centigrade degrees by 9, divide by 5, add 32.

To convert Fahrenheit into Centigrade: Subtract 32 from degrees of Fahrenheit and multiply by 5, then divide by 9.

	Fahrenheit	Centigrade
Water freezes	32°	0°
Water boils	212°	100°
Absolute zero	−459.6°	−273.1°

CONVERSION TABLE FOR COMMON U.S. AND METRIC MEASUREMENTS
Linear
1 inch = 2.54 centimeters
1 foot = 30.48 centimeters
1 yard = .914 meter
1 mile = 1.610 kilometers

1 millimeter = .03937 inch
1 centimeter = .3937 inch
1 meter = 3.2808 feet = 1.0936 yards
1 kilometer = .621 mile

*Centigrade also known as "Celsius"

Area
1 acre = .4047 hectare   1 hectare = 2.4711 acres

Weight
1 ounce = 28.3495 grams   1 gram = .035 ounce
1 pound = .4536 kilograms   1 kilogram = 2.204 pounds
1 ton = 907.18 kilograms   1 metric ton = 1.1023 tons

Volume
1 ounce = 29.58 milliliters   1 milliliter = .0348 ounce
1 quart = .9464 liters   1 liter = 1.0567 quarts
1 gallon = 3.7854 liters   1 liter = .2642 gallon
1 cubic inch = 16.39 cubic centimeters   1 cubic centimeter = .0610 cubic inch
1 cubic foot = .0283 cubic meter   1 cubic meter = 35.325 cubic feet
                                      1 cubic meter = 1.3080 cubic yards
1 cubic yard = .7646 cubic meter

Fever Chart

Fahrenheit	Centigrade
105°	40.5°
104°	40°
103°	39.4°
102°	38.8°
101°	38.3°
100°	37.7°
98.6°	37° (normal)
97°	36.1°

Weather Chart

Fahrenheit	Centigrade
110°	43°
100°	37.8°
90°	32.2°
80°	26.7°
70°	21.1°
60°	15.6°
50°	10°
40°	4.4°
32°	0°
20°	−6.7°
10°	−12.2°
0°	−17.8°
−10°	−23.3°
−20°	−28.9°

MILES/KILOMETERS FOR MOTORISTS

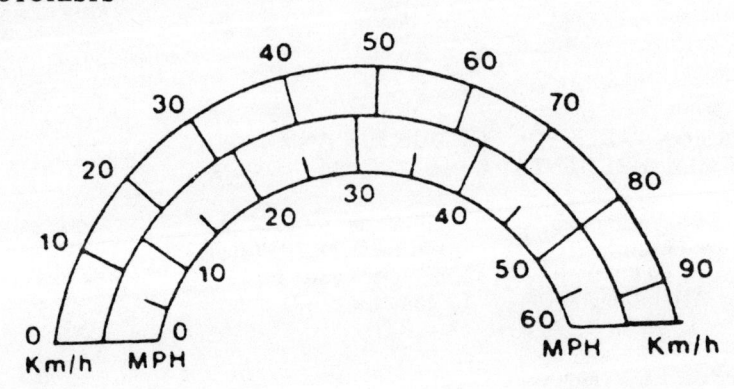

REFERENCES

Brown, Ross, M.D. *Ultrasonography Basic Principles and Clinical Applications*. St. Louis, Missouri: Warren H. Green, 1975.

Bryan, Glenda J. *Diagnostic Radiography*. Baltimore: Williams and Wilkins, 1970.

Burkhart, Roger, L., Ph.D. *Diagnostic Radiology Quality Assurance Catalog*. Rockville, Maryland: U.S. Department of Health, Education and Welfare (HEW), HEW Publication (FDA) 77-8028, 1977.

Bushong, Stewart C. *Radiologic Science for Technologists*. St. Louis, Missouri: C. V. Mosby, 1975.

Cahoon, John B., R. T., FASRT. *Formulating X-ray Techniques*. Durham, North Carolina: Duke University, 1970.

Christensen, Edward E., Thomas S. Curry III, and James Nunnally. *An Introduction to the Physics of Diagnostic Radiology*. Philadelphia: Lea & Febiger, 1973.

Culverwell, Robert H. *The Relationship of Conventional Medical X-ray Film to Silver and Non-silver Image Recording Media*. GAF Corporation, 1975.

Dietz, K. *The X-ray Tube in Diagnostic Application*. Erlangen, Germany: Siemens Aktiengesellschaft Medical Engineering Group.

Etter, Lewis, E., B.S., M.D., F.A.C.R. *Glossary of Words and Phases Used in Radiology, Nuclear Medicine and Ultrasound*. Springfield, Illinois: Charles C. Thomas, 1970.

Files, Glenn W. (ed). "Body Section Radiography." in *Medical Radiographic Technic*. Revised by William L. Bloom, Jr., John L. Hollenbach, R.T., James A. Morgan, R.T. and John B. Thomas, R.T. 2d. Ed. Springfield, Illinois: Charles C. Thomas, 1962.

Forsythe, C. W. *Service Manual DXR 750-II*. Milwaukee, Wisconsin: X-ray Unit Medical Systems SM A0642D.

Grigg, E. R. N., M.D. *The Trail of the Invisible Light*. Springfield, Illinois: Charles C. Thomas, 1965.

Halliday, David and Robert Resnick. *Fundamentals of Physics*. New York: John Wiley, 1970.

Jacobi, Charles A. and Don Q. Paris. *Textbook of Radiologic Technology*. St. Louis, Missouri: C. V. Mosby, 1972.

Just Enough Logarithms for Sensitometry. Eastman Kodak Company, 1961-63.

Laubenberger, Theodor van. *Leitfaden der medizinischen Roentgentechnik*. Köln-Lövenich, Germany: Deutscher Äzte-Berieg GmbH, 1975.

Markus, John. *Electronics and Nucleonics Dictionary*. New York: McGraw-Hill, 1966.

Medical Service Radiologic Technology. Department of the Air Force, the Army, and the Navy, 1974.

Morgan, James A., R.T. *The Art and Science of Medical Radiography*. St. Louis, Missouri: Charles C. Thomas, 1972.

Myers, Patricia A., R.T.(R), FASRT. *An Introduction to Radiographic Technique*. New York: Praeger, 1980.

Myers, Patricia A., R.T.(R), FASRT. *Complete Technical Glossary for Radiologic Technologists*. Pittsburgh, Pennsylvania: Radiological Textbooks, 1973.

Rich, J. E. *Intensified Fluoroscopy in the Radiology Department*. General Electric, 1980.

Rich, J. E. *Television in the Radiology Department*. General Electric, 1969.

Riemann, Mathew. "A New Generation of X-ray Generators." in *Applied Radiology*. Los Angeles, California: Barrington, November/December 1975.

Ross, John A. and R. W. Galloway. *A Handbook of Radiography*. Philadelphia: J. B. Lippincott, 1963.

Saxton, H. M. and Basil Strickland. *Practical Procedures in Diagnostic Radiology*. New York: Grune & Stratton, 1972.

Schulz, R. J., Ph.D. *Diagnostic X-ray Physics*. New York: GAF, 1977.

Seemann, Herman E. *Physical and Photographic Principles of Medical Radiography*. New York: John Wiley, 1968.

"Sensitometric Properties of X-ray Film." Eastman Kodak Company,

Selman, Joseph, M.D. *Fundamentals of X-ray and Radium Physics*. St. Louis, Missouri: Charles C. Thomas, 1977.

Sprawls, Perry Jr. *The Physical Principles of Diagnostic Radiology*. Baltimore, Maryland: University Park Press, 1977.

Stanton, Leonard, M.S., F.A.C.R. *Basic Medical Radiation Physics*. New York: Appleton-Century-Crofts, 1969.

Stevens, Matthew and Robert I. Phillips. *Comprehensive Review for the Radiologic Technologist*. St. Louis, Missouri: C. V. Mosby, 1968.

Ter-Pogossian, Michel M. *The Physical Aspects of Diagnostic Radiology*. New York: Hoeber Medical Division, Harper & Row, 1969.

The Fundamentals of Radiography. Eastman Kodak Company, 1968.

van der Plaat, G. J. *Medical X-ray Technique*. New York: The Macmillan Press, LTD., 1972.

Westra, D. "History of Tomography," *Modern Thin-Section Tomography*. Edited by A. Barrett, M.D. and G. Valvassori. Springfield, Illinois: Charles C. Thomas, 1973.